Walk the Weight Away!

Walk the Weight Away!

The Easiest Weight-Loss Plan Ever!

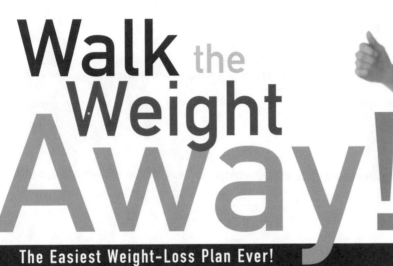

Andrew Flach & RoseMarie Alfieri

Photographs by Peter Field Peck

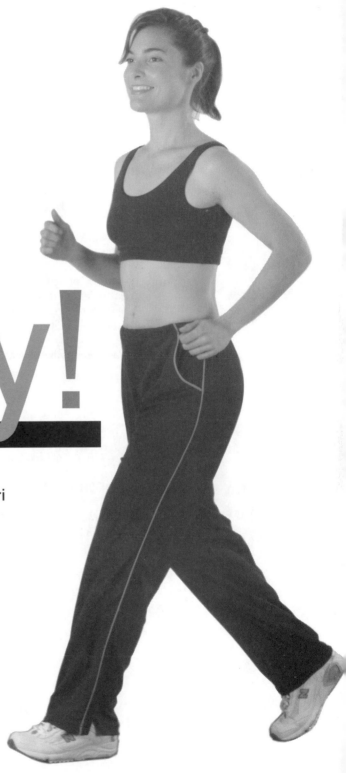

Healthy Living Books
New York • London

Join the *Walk the Weight Away!* on-line community:

- **Find out more** about walking for weight-loss.
- **Get answers** to your walking questions from our fitness pros.
- **Learn how to start** your own walking club.
- **Sign up** to receive a free Healthy Living e-newsletter.
- **Receive special offers** on fitness books and products.
  And more!
  Visit today at www.walktheweightaway.com

Text and photos © 2003 by Healthy Living Books

Workout apparel shown on pages 107 to 134 provided by New Balance. To find local retailers that carry New Balance products, consumers can call 1-800-253-SHOE or visit www.newbalance.com

Healthy Living Books
Hatherleigh Press
5-22 46th Avenue, Suite 200
Long Island City, NY 11101

www.healthylivingbooks.com

Library of Congress Cataloging-in-Publication Data

Flach, Andrew, 1961-
Walk the weight away! : the easiest weight-loss program ever—for fast results without diets, pills, or surgery! / Andrew Flach & RoseMarie Alfieri ; photographs by Peter Field.
   p. cm.
ISBN 1-57826-138-4 (pbk. : alk. paper)
1. Weight loss. 2. Walking. I. Alfieri, RoseMarie. II. Title.
RM222.2.F526 2003
613.2'5—dc22

                                        2003016592

Information included in this book is for your general knowledge only and is not intended as a substitute for the advice or care of medical professionals. Please consult your physician or other healthcare professional before starting any new physical fitness program.

All Healthy Living Books titles are available for special promotions and premiums. For more information, please contact the manager of our Special Sales department at 800-528-2550.

ISBN 1-57826-138-4

Cover & Interior Design by Tai Blanche
Exercise Photos by Peter Field Peck

Printed in Canada
10 9 8 7 6 5 4 3 2 1

Table of Contents

Part II: *Walk the Weight Away!* Day-by-Day

Walk
the
Weight
Away!

Introduction
Welcome to *Walk the Weight Away!*

Do you have a few (or many) pounds that you want to lose? Do you enjoy walking and hope to start a regular walking program? Are you ready to change your life for the better? We believe that *Walk the Weight Away!* will help you do just that. We've put together a walking and eating program that you not only can live with, but that will enhance your life. If you follow the guidelines in this book, you will walk your way to a happy, healthier, lighter you in just a few weeks time. Can a walking program really do that? It certainly can.

A couple of years ago Linda, a good friend of mine from my high school days, called me for some fitness advice. She was frustrated because over the years 10 extra pounds gradually had crept up on her. As a working mother of two young girls in her mid-thirties, her life was busy to say the least, and she didn't have time to join a gym and spend hours a week exercising. Moreover, Linda hates to exercise—always has. "The only thing I really like to do is walk," she said, almost apologetically. Bingo!

I devised a walking program for Linda that fit into her schedule. She started walking through her neighborhood in the evenings after supper. Linda enjoyed that time of day because it was quiet and peaceful. She took the time that she normally would have spent watching a sitcom and instead went outside and walked. In addition to her walking program, Linda began to be more careful about her diet, watching portion sizes and making sure that she ate healthful, nutrient-dense foods. Within a couple of months, Linda had lost the 10 pounds. She was ecstatic. She could not believe that she had achieved such great results, with really such minimal effort. Not only that, but she truly looked forward to her daily walks. They became her "me"

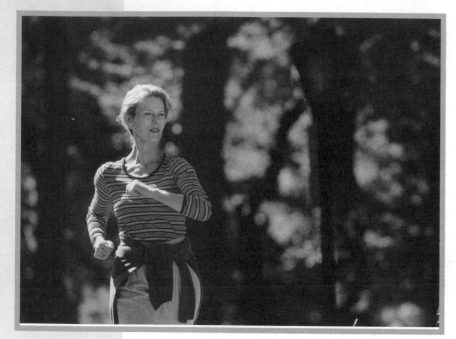

time—time during which she could let her mind roam free as her legs took her closer and closer to her weight goals. Linda continues to walk regularly today. It truly has become an integral part of her life.

Linda discovered that something that comes as naturally as walking can have tremendous health and fitness benefits. Like many people she had been led to believe that the only way to lose weight was to join an expensive gym and spend lots of time performing vigorous activities while starving yourself. She couldn't imagine that doing an activity that she enjoyed—walking—could help her lose weight and feel better.

In *Walk the Weight Away!*, we provide you with an eating and walking program that you can easily tailor to fit your life and which will help you reach your weight loss goals. More importantly, this is a sensible program that you can maintain over your lifetime. It is not a fad. It is not based on losing a lot of weight quickly or spending hours at the gym sweating. It requires two things: that you walk and start paying attention to what you eat. Sound doable?

Walk
the
Weight
Away!

How to Use This Book

This book is unique in that it functions both as a guide *and* as a workbook. In Part I, we discuss the research behind the weight-loss and health benefits of walking and then look at the "hows" and "whys" of weight-loss. We also include basic nutritional information and sample recipes to make it as easy as possible for you to eat well as you lose weight. Because adopting a weight loss and exercise program can be a big lifestyle change for people, we look at the psychology behind behavior change and give you the advice you'll need in order to successfully make these changes to your new positive way of life.

You'll also learn everything you need to know about gearing up for your walk and about the basics of exercise, in particular how aerobic conditioning helps your heart to pump better, and your body to shed fat. We'll also talk about strength training and flexibility, and why it's important for you to incorporate these pillars of fitness into your workouts.

In Part II your daily walking program is present- ed step by step. You don't have to think about anything, just follow the guidelines for the day. This program is progressive, meaning that as time goes by you make it a little more challenging by adding intensity, time, or distance. In this section you will find workbook pages in which to record your daily walking and exercise routine, and keep track of your success. In addition, we provide strength training and stretching routines for you to add to your walking pro- gram as you grow more proficient. We do this because research has shown that strength training improves overall body tone and raises your resting metabolism (which allows you to burn more calories at rest). You will also find eight weeks' worth of food diaries in which to record your daily eating habits. Recording your eating and walking information will help you monitor your progress and determine what changes you should make to reach your goals.

Are you ready to begin your walk toward a slimmer, healthier you? Turn the page and let's begin.

Introduction
Welcome to
Walk the Weight Away!

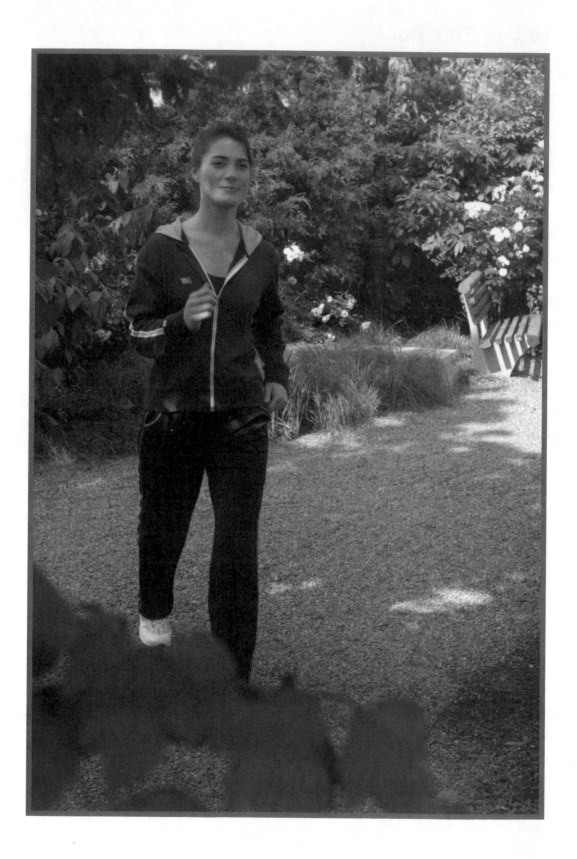

Part I

The
Walk the Weight Away!
Program

Chapter 1

Why Walk?

You may have selected this book because you want to lose weight and walking appeals to you as a mode of exercise. Even if you aren't thrilled by the idea of exercising, at least you can see yourself adopting a walking program. Walking is the most popular exercise of choice among Americans. There are several reasons for this. Walking is the most natural of all exercises, something we've been doing ever since we learned how to do it. No one had to teach us to walk; it is a natural part of our physical development. We crawl; we walk. Walking also doesn't require a financial commitment, like joining a gym does—it's free.

Because it doesn't require a lot of gear, and can be done virtually anywhere and anytime, it's also the most convenient way to carve activity into your daily life. You can walk in the morning before you get ready for work, during your lunch hour, or in the evenings. You can walk indoors or outside. Walking also offers a great deal of variety as a form of exercise. For example, you can vary the speed of your walking, the route of your walk, or the terrain (flat ground, hills, or a combination). Varying your routine will help keep your walking program interesting and challenging.

Walking to Lose Weight

Walking is a great exercise for weight loss. The number of calories you burn depends on the distance, speed, and intensity of your walk. Generally speaking, an average-size person burns approximately 90 to 100 calories for every mile walked. If you walk 2 miles a day you'll burn about 200 calories.

The Top 10 Reasons to Walk

1. It's the most natural way to exercise—most of us have been doing it since we were toddlers.

2. It's the very best way to start an exercise program. Even if you've never exercised, you'll be able to walk.

3. It doesn't cost a cent.

4. Your walk time is for you to enjoy. You can meditate, listen to your favorite music, or solve problems—whatever helps you keep on walking.

5. You can walk alone or with family and friends.

6. It's safe. It's almost impossible to get injured while walking.

7. It's easy to adapt to your fitness level. Start out slowly and gradually build to a fast, fat-burning pace.

8. Walking improves muscle tone—especially around the butt and hips.

9. It promotes an overall sense of wellness. It's nice knowing you're doing something good for yourself.

10. It's portable: You can do it anywhere—at home, at work, on vacation.

While you don't have to walk fast to burn calories, your walk should be on the brisk side (about 15 minutes per mile) for health benefits and to make the exercise more of an aerobic activity. However, if you are just starting a walking program, go easy, and slowly work up to the 15-minute pace.

Of course the longer, faster, and harder you walk, the more calories you will burn and the more weight you will lose. But don't overdo it. When people begin a new workout program, they sometimes get caught up in the

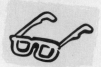

Walking is the most natural of all exercises, something we've been doing ever since we were toddlers. And the best part? It's free.

13

excitement of their new activity and are tempted to do a lot at once. Consequently, they often end up burning out because they do too much too soon. The most important determinant of your long-term weight-loss success is your ability to make your walking program a routine part of your life.

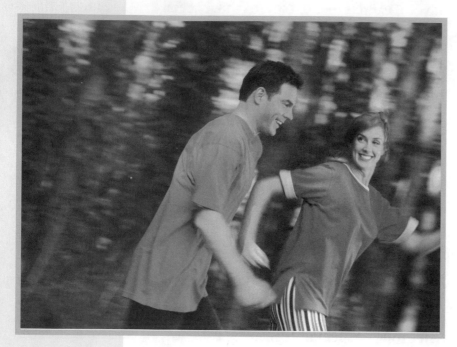

Weight-loss is just one of many good health-related reasons to start a walking program. In fact, a study of 13,000 people, conducted over eight years, found that people who walk for 30 minutes a day are at much lower risk of premature death than those who don't exercise regularly.

Another study, one of postmenopausal women, found that those who walked regularly were less likely to have heart disease; in addition, they had fewer hospitalizations, surgeries, and falls. Let's take a look at the specific health-related benefits of walking.

Cardiovascular Health

Research has shown that walking, like all cardiovascular exercise, can reduce blood cholesterol, lower blood pressure, and increase cardiovascular endurance, enabling your heart to pump blood to your cells more efficiently. Recently, a large study of 44,452 people found that walking reduced risk for cardiovascular disease by 23 percent. This study also discovered that walking pace was related to the protection from cardiovascular disease more than the distance walked, with those who walked at greater speeds and intensities getting more protection. In other words, the faster and harder you walk, the greater the benefit for your heart.

Bone Protection

If you don't get much exercise, beginning a walking program can help protect your bones from osteoporosis—a prevalent disease characterized by the loss of bone density. The disease is most common among post-menopausal women, who comprise 80 percent of all cases, and it leads to susceptibility to fracture. A review of several studies by researchers from the Massachusetts General Hospital Institute of Health Professions in Boston found that sedentary women who walked increased their bone mass by 2 percent.

Walking can help initially boost your bone density because it forces your bones to support weight (this is called a weight-bearing exercise). However, your bones must be progressively challenged in order to maintain their density. With time you will also need to incorporate other weight-bearing activity, such as strength training, for maximum protection against osteoporosis.

Psychological Health

There is also evidence that physical activity can help improve your mood and alleviate stress and depression. While exercising, your body stimulates neurotransmitters such as endorphins, which help you feel good. Their production helps alleviate anxiety and also allows your body to relax. It is thought that one exercise session can generate 90 to 120 minutes of relaxation response. On top of that very chemical reaction, there's always the satisfaction that comes from knowing you've done something good for your body.

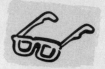

Not only will walking improve your physical health, but it also improves your mental health, reducing stress and helping you relax.

15

Losing Weight

nergy. Energy. Energy. To understand how you can lose weight, you need to think about just one word: Energy. The energy your body takes in from food and drink (in the form of calories) is necessary for several reasons:

1. Your body needs a lot of energy simply to keep you alive, even if you are doing nothing at all. It takes a lot of work to keep your heart pumping blood to your cells, and to sustain other involuntary processes that keep us alive.

2. You need even more energy to perform activities such as sitting, walking, doing chores, exercising, and the like.

3. Finally, your body requires additional energy for your digestive system to break down the fats, proteins, and carbohydrates you eat. This energy is called the *thermic effect* of a meal and actually accounts for 10 percent of all your daily caloric needs. Bet you never thought that you actually burn calories *after* eating.

The total of these three factors: your energy requirements at rest, for activity and exercise, and to digest food, all add up to the total number of calories that you need *each day*. If you consume that exact number of calories you will be in a state of *energy balance,* meaning that the energy you're taking in is equal to the energy that you're expending. Consequently, you will neither gain nor lose weight.

If, on the other hand, you consistently consume more calories than your body requires, you will gain weight.

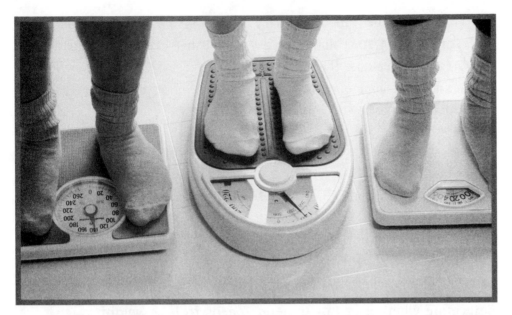

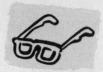

If you want to lose weight, you must consume fewer calories than your body burns. It's that simple.

See where we're going with this? To lose weight, you need to consume fewer calories than your body burns. Now, there are safe ways and unsafe ways to go about losing weight. To understand more, let's talk about metabolism.

Resting Metabolic Rate

Resting metabolic rate (RMR) refers to the calories (or energy) that your body expends when you're at rest. RMR is the metabolic rate that people talk about when they complain that they have a slow metabolism. Your RMR is calculated first thing in the morning, after fasting and having at least eight hours of sleep. RMR indicates how much lean mass you have, as opposed to fat; the higher your RMR, the higher your percentage of lean body mass. This explains why people who are more muscular have higher resting metabolisms—muscle requires more energy than fat.

This also explains why if you lose fat and gain lean body mass you will burn more calories at rest than you did previously. In other words, after exercising away your unwanted fat, and perhaps adding some strength training to your program, you will actually burn more calories doing nothing! We'll talk more about this in the section on strength training. For now, back to diet.

In general, your RMR requirements represent the *minimum number of calories that you should consume each day* (because, remember that RMR is

Chapter 2
Losing Weight

related to the proper functioning of your vital systems). Most women have RMRs of at least 1,200 calories per day; men usually fall somewhere around 1,500 calories per day. Therefore, in order to lose weight safely, without interfering with your body's metabolic needs, most people shouldn't eat fewer than 1,200 or 1,500 calories a day.

BMI

You may be familiar with the term BMI. It stands for body mass index and it's a ratio of your weight in kilograms to your height in meters squared. Some weight-loss experts use the resulting number to determine whether or not someone needs to lose weight.

Ideally, your BMI should fall between 19 and 25. If it is over 25, you may be overweight; if it is over 30, you may be obese. BMI estimates and height / weight charts provide easy reference, though they are somewhat flawed. Neither tells you how much of your weight is from fat and how much is made up of lean body mass (muscle, bones, connective tissues). We know that muscle weighs more than fat, so it stands to reason that a very fit person with a great deal of muscle may have a high BMI. However, for most of the non-weightlifting population BMI and height / weight charts are reasonable starting points when determining your healthy weight.

If you want to determine your own BMI (and don't want to do all the math), use the chart below.

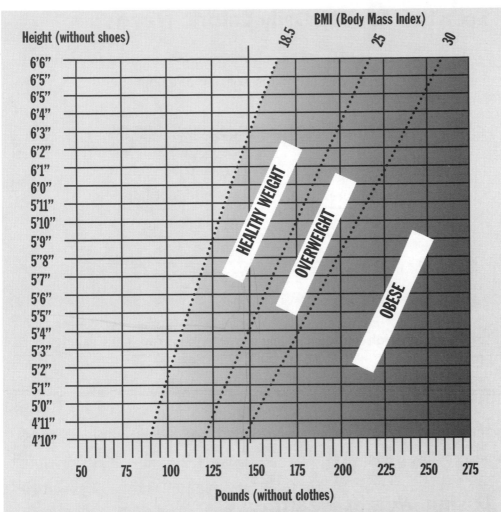

BMI (Body Mass Index)

Height (without shoes)

6'6"
6'5"
6'5"
6'4"
6'3"
6'2"
6'1"
6'0"
5'11"
5'10"
5'9"
5"8"
5'7"
5'6"
5'5"
5'4"
5'3"
5'2"
5'1"
5'0"
4'11"
4'10"

18.5   25   30

HEALTHY WEIGHT   OVERWEIGHT   OBESE

50   75   100   125   150   175   200   225   250   275

Pounds (without clothes)

BMI measures weight in relation to height. The BMI ranges shown above are for adults. They are not exact ranges of healthy and unhealthy weights. However, they show that health risk increases at higher levels of overweight and obesity. Even within the healthy BMI range, weight gains can carry health risks for adults.

Directions: Find your weight on the bottom of the graph. Go straight up from that point until you come to the line that matches your height. Then look to find your weight group.

Healthy Weight: BMI from 18.5 up to 25 refers to a healthy weight.
Overweight: BMI from 25 up to 30 refers to overweight.
Obese: BMI 30 or higher refers to obesity. Obese persons are also overweight.

Chapter 2
Losing Weight

So What Are My Daily Caloric Needs?

Here's how to estimate the number of calories you need to consume to maintain your current weight (that is, not lose or gain).

ESTIMATING DAILY CALORIE NEEDS

If you are . .	Multiply Your Weight (in pounds) by:
Sedentary	11
More Active	12 or 13
Very Active	15, 16, or 17

Let's say you weigh 160 pounds and are sedentary. Your daily caloric needs would be:

160 x 11 = 1,760 calories per day

That means you can consume (about) 1,760 calories each day and neither gain nor lose weight.

Losing Weight Healthfully

You can use this information about your current caloric needs to figure out how many calories you should take in to lose weight.

Let's take an example of a sedentary adult woman who we'll call Sara. She weighs 150 pounds now, but her goal weight is 130 pounds. Sara currently needs to consume 1,650 calories each day to maintain her weight (150 x 11). If she consumes fewer than 1,650 calories each day, she will lose weight. Sara can safely lose weight by cutting back her current caloric intake by about 300 calories a day and doing enough exercise to burn an additional 200 calories.

This approach will provide Sara with a daily calorie deficit of 500 calories. Since 1 pound of fat equals approximately 3,500 calories, Sara will lose about one pound a week. A weight-loss rate of 1 to 2 pounds per week is considered safe and recommended by most experts. Such a slow and steady approach ensures that your body gets the proper amount and variety of nutrients, and that weight loss is from fat and not water (beware of quick loss diets that promise a 5-pound weight loss in one week. Most of that weight loss is certain to be water).

Most important, research has shown that people who adopt slower, consistent weight-loss programs based on cutting back calories and exercising not only attain their weight goals, they are able to keep the weight off for years. Remember that children's story about the hare and the tortoise? The tortoise challenges the hare to a race—the hare, haughty as can be because he is so much faster than the tortoise gets cocky and lazy. In the end, the tortoise, with determination and consistent effort, wins the race. It is the same way with diet and weight loss: Slow and steady wins the race.

To determine the calories that you will need to cut to lose weight, first calculate the number of calories your body needs to maintain your current weight. Then, subtract between 300 and 500 calories. The resulting number represents your daily caloric allowance from food. Remember that you also will be burning calories in your walking program. The exact number of calories will vary depending upon your weight and the speed and distance you walk, and will probably range anywhere from 100 to 400 calories per workout (see Chart).

How much weight you decide to lose in total depends on your goals—do you want to be more healthy, or do you want to fit into a particular outfit that you wore only last year? To get a sense of what constitutes a normal healthy weight for you, check a height / weight table (see table). Better yet, determine your body mass index (BMI). However, bear in mind that these numbers provide general guidelines on desirable weights and that optimal weights may vary from person to person. One thing is true for everyone: It is important that you make your weight-loss goal both realistic and attainable. Saying you want

Calories Burned Per Minute of Walking

Body Weight (lb)	2.0 mph	2.5 mph	3.0 mph	3.5 mph	4.0 mph	4.5 mph	5.0 mph
110	2.1	2.4	2.8	3.1	4.1	5.2	6.6
120	2.3	2.6	3.0	3.4	4.4	5.6	7.2
130	2.5	2.9	3.2	3.6	4.8	6.1	7.8
140	2.7	3.1	3.?	3.9	5.2	6.6	8.4
150	2.8	3.3	3.7	4.2	5.6	7.0	9.0
160	3.0	3.5	4.0	4.5	5.9	7.5	9.6
170	3.2	3.7	4.2	4.8	6.3	8.0	10.2
180	3.4	4.0	4.5	5.0	6.7	8.4	10.8
190	3.7	4.2	4.7	5.3	7.0	8.9	11.4
200	3.8	4.4	5.0	5.6	7.4	9.4	12.6
210	4.0	4.6	5.2	5.9	7.8	9.9	12.6
220	4.2	4.8	5.5	6.2	8.2	10.3	13.2

Source: Franks D., & Howley, E. (1992). *Health Fitness Instructor's Handbook*

to lose 20 pounds in two weeks is not only unrealistic, it is dangerous and probably unattainable. This is why experts recommend adopting a diet/exercise plan that will enable you lose from one to two pounds each week.

Nutrition Basics

Since diet is integral to weight loss, we'll talk a bit here about the basics of nutrition. Food, in the form of nutrients, is the fuel that drives your body. There are four major macronutrients: proteins, carbohydrates, fats, and water. In addition, your body needs minerals and vitamins to function properly and

Walk
the
Weight
Away!

prevent disease. Think of all nutrients as energy sources your body can go to for fuel, each of a different type, each equally important. Let's look at what the macronutrients do.

Proteins are the building blocks of life, and are made up of amino acids. Your hair, skin, and muscles, are all formed from protein. Protein also makes enzymes and hormones that regulate your body's systems, fights disease as a component of antibodies, and provides energy. About 80 percent of all proteins are manufactured by your body. The rest must be obtained through the foods you eat. Animal proteins—from meat, fish, and chicken—are considered complete proteins because they contain all the amino acids you require from food. Proteins from vegetables, nuts, and beans are inadequate individually and must be carefully combined in order to form complete proteins. This is why vegetarians are at risk for protein deficiency. *Your protein intake should be about 12 to 20 percent of your daily caloric intake.*

Carbohydrates are your body's best source of energy. There are two classes of carbs: simple carbs, which include fruits and sweets, and complex carbs, which include the more dense foods like whole grain breads, brown rice, and vegetables. In general, it is wise to consume much more of the colorful and complex carbs—which are much more nutritious—and fewer of the simple white carbs, such as white rice, sugar, and white bread. While many fruits are simple carbs, they provide a wealth of vitamins that are vital to your health. *The American Dietetic Association suggests that carbs comprise 55 to 60 percent of your daily caloric intake.*

Carbohydrates have been much maligned lately. Proponents of popular high-protein, high-fat diets maintain that over consumption of carbohydrates leads to weight gain because too many carbohydrates in the blood can lead to a pre-diabetes condition. These diets theorize that when you have this condition (known as insulin resistance) your body, unable to process the extra sugar in your blood, will store it as fat. Is this true?

Yes it is true that excessive consumption of carbohydrates, especially the simple carbs, can lead to glucose intolerance. The important distinction is the word "excessive." During the eighties, the high-carb / low-fat craze encouraged the thinking that eating loads of carbohydrates would prevent weight gain. People often consume too much rice, pasta, or other white carbs that quickly break down into sugar. In addition, they ate fat-free cookies by the box, thinking that, because they were fat-free, they were "safe." In fact, those fat-

Contrary to current popular belief, there's no such thing as a bad nutrient: carbohydrates, protein—and yes, even fat—all perform important jobs in your body.

Chapter 2
Losing Weight

free cookies were loaded with simple sugar. In the end, people consumed more calories than they were burning and got fatter (remember weight maintenance is all about energy balance).

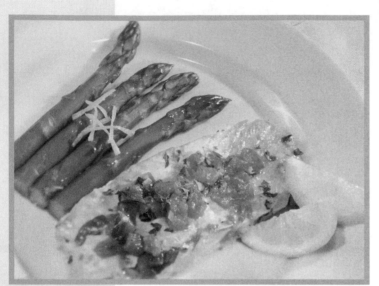

You see it doesn't matter whether those extra calories come from fat, protein, or carbs—all extra calories are stored as fat. Portion control, and eating the right percentage of each nutrient within a total daily caloric guideline, is the key to enjoying all your nutrients, carbs included.

Fat serves important functions: It is a great source of energy for many of your body's functions and it helps in the absorption of the fat-soluble vitamins A, D, E, and K. In addition, because fat is more energy-dense than carbs or proteins (fat packs 9 calories in every gram, while one gram of carbs and proteins only contains 4 calories), you can feel full while eating less.

There are definitely good and bad fats. The bad fats are the ones that come primarily from animal sources—the saturated fats. These fats can clog arteries and lead to heart disease. Saturated fat should comprise less than 10 percent of your diet. The good fats are the monounsaturated and polyunsaturated fats found in many vegetable oils, olive oil, canola oil, and nuts. Beware of vegetable oils that have been hydrogenated (this will be indicated on the food label). Hydrogenated oils are very unhealthy because they turn into trans fatty acids, which not only raise levels of bad cholesterol, but also lower the levels of good cholesterol.

Other good fats are essential fatty acids (EFAs), such as the Omega-3 fats found in fatty fish like mackerel, tuna, and salmon. EFAs are vital for many of your body's functions, including growth and hormone development. In addition, increased consumption of EFAs has been found to decrease the risk of heart disease. In fact, the American Heart Association recently revised its dietary guidelines to include the recommendation that we eat at least two servings of fatty fish each week. *Overall, fat should comprise no more than 25 to 30 percent of your daily caloric intake.*

The Fat-Free Myth

For too long, we've bought into the myth that fat is evil and that to lose weight all we had to do was cut fat from our diets. But substituting non-fat or low-fat products for fats hasn't lead to successful weight loss. Why? Here are the facts about fats.

FACT: Fat-free does not equal calorie-free. Many non-fat and low-fat foods contain loads of sugar, which can significantly increase their caloric content. In addition, people tend to eat larger portions of fat-free food, thereby increasing the number of calories consumed.

FACT: Fat satiates. You generally feel more full after eating food with fat than when eating the fat-free or low-fat alternative. That's one reason people tend to eat larger portions of fat-free and low-fat foods.

FACT: You need some fat. This one is difficult for many people to accept, but it's true. Fat is a major nutrient and is vital for proper growth and development, as well as overall maintenance of good health. Certain vitamins (A, D, E, and K) are soluble only in fat. The *Walk the Weight Away!* nutrition plan, which is based on the Food Guide Pyramid, recommends that approximately 25 to 30 percent of your daily diet come from fat.

If you wait until you're thirsty to take a drink, you're already dehydrated. Your best bet is to drink small amounts of water through-out the day.

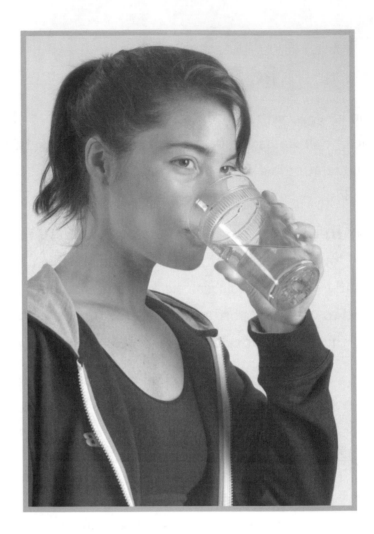

Drink Up!

Your body needs more water than any other nutrient. Seventy-five per-cent of our body weight comes from water. A component of all cells, water transports various nutrients to our cells and removes toxins. It also provides moisture for our respiratory system and aids in digestion. Most of us, how-ever, do not drink nearly enough water. Thirst is your body's way of saying you are already dehydrated. Experts suggest consuming three quarts of water a day, which can seem daunting. The best way to drink water is in small amounts throughout the day and with your meals. When you exercise, you should drink 8 to 12 ounces before beginning your workout and then an additional 4 to 8 ounces during your exercise session.

Fast Facts about Water

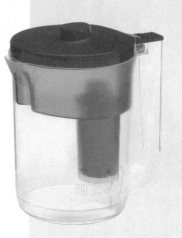

Did you know that...

- Water makes up 55 to 75 percent of our total body weight. That means that there is more water in our bodies than any other substance.

- We can't live without water. It transports nutrients throughout the body, aids in digestion and the expulsion of waste products, helps protect organs, tissues, and joints, and plays an essential role in controlling body temperature.

- We lose approximately 10 glasses of water each day through our activities and bodily functions. Adults should drink at least eight to 12 glasses of water throughout the day to replenish the supply of water in their bodies. You should drink even more during hot weather, while you exercise, when you have a headache, diarrhea or fever, and if you are pregnant or nursing a baby.

To make sure you are getting enough water each day:

- Bring a bottle of water with you whenever you go out, particularly during a heat wave and when you exercise.

- Drink a glass of water with every meal, in addition to the other beverages you may consume.

- Always keep a full container of water in your refrigerator. Drink a glass of water before you head for bed, and another as soon as you rise in the morning.

- Every time you pass a drinking fountain, stop and drink some water.

- Drink water while you prepare your meals and as you relax in front of the television.

- Above all, make sure that the water you drink is clean and healthy. Water filtration pitchers are a simple, inexpensive solution for reducing odor, sediment and contaminants that can be found in tap water.

Here's a tip: Keep a pitcher of ice-cold water in the fridge. A water filtration pitcher, like this Brita model, keeps the water pure and is a less expensive solution than buying bottled water.

27

Let the Pyramid Guide You

The Department of Agriculture's Food Guide Pyramid provides a good guideline for the variety of foods you should eat, and suggested servings for each food group per day. The pyramid, shown below, is broken into six food groups: grains, vegetables and fruits, dairy products, proteins, fats and sweets. Note that according to the pyramid, most of your foods should come from carbohydrates in the form of cereals, breads, rice and pasta. But don't let the 6 to 11 servings fool you into thinking you can eat a ton of these foods. You might be surprised to learn that a serving of pasta is only one-half a cup. Consume one large bowl of pasta and you can see how you could easily eat through 4 or 5 servings of your entire daily allowance for grains in one meal.

Currently, there is talk among experts that the Food Guide Pyramid should be revised to differentiate between so-called "good" and "bad" fats, as well as distinguishing more nutritious carbs from those that are more likely to lead to glucose intolerance. Such a revision could help people make more informed decisions about what foods they eat based on their nutritional values. We suggest using the pyramid to ensure your diet contains a varied and well-proportioned mix of nutrients.

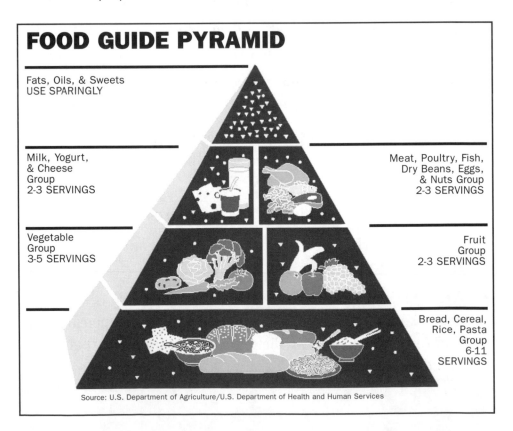

FOOD GUIDE PYRAMID

Fats, Oils, & Sweets
USE SPARINGLY

Milk, Yogurt,
& Cheese
Group
2-3 SERVINGS

Meat, Poultry, Fish,
Dry Beans, Eggs,
& Nuts Group
2-3 SERVINGS

Vegetable
Group
3-5 SERVINGS

Fruit
Group
2-3 SERVINGS

Bread, Cereal,
Rice, Pasta
Group
6-11
SERVINGS

Source: U.S. Department of Agriculture/U.S. Department of Health and Human Services

Pay Heed to Portion Sizes

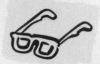

Do the portion sizes recommended by the Food Guide Pyramid have you confused? Is that huge hamburger that nearly takes up your entire plate at your local pub really one serving of meat? Here's the surprising truth:

- 1 serving of breads or grains is equal to 1 slice of bread or ½ cup cooked rice or pasta!

- 1 serving of fruit is 1 small fruit.

- 1 serving of vegetables is usually ½ cup.

- 1 serving of meat is approximately the size of the palm of your hand (about 3 or 4 ounces).

Read food labels carefully. You'll often find that a bag of chips or box of cookies contains several servings.

Keep a careful eye on the number of servings in your favorite packaged foods. A small bag of chips may contain as many as three servings.

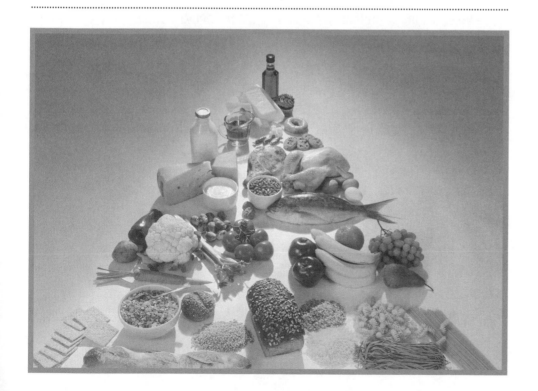

Reading Food Labels

Learning how to properly interpret the information presented on a food label gives you a valuable nutrition tool. The ingredients listed first are the ones present in the highest concentrations by weight. Too often those ingredients are sugar and sodium. Try to buy foods that have healthy ingredients front and center.

The serving sizes listed on labels can also be misleading. A small bag of potato chips may list "150 calories per serving" and you think "that's not so bad," but you need to carefully read how many servings the bag contains, which can often be two or three. So, if you eat all the chips in a bag that contains three servings, you've actually consumed 450 calories. Not so good.

Finally, it is helpful to know how to convert the nutrients presented on the label in grams to calories in order to determine how much (energy-wise) of each individual nutrient you would be eating in a serving.

Carbohydrates:	1 gram equals 4 calories
Proteins:	1 gram equals 4 calories
Fats:	1 gram equals 9 calories

When reading labels pay particular attention to the amount of cholesterol and sodium listed. You might be surprised at how many low-fat and low-calorie foods contain very high levels of sodium (healthy adults should aim for a total intake of no more than 2400 milligrams per day.) When reading the ingredient list check to see whether the food contains any saturated or hydrogenated oils; if it does, you may want to avoid it since hydrogenated foods contain the unhealthy and potentially harmful trans-fatty acids.

In the last chapter, you learned how to estimate your daily caloric needs, and how to create a calorie deficit to lose weight. The information you have learned about nutrition is important to your health and is the key to achieving your weight-loss goals. In the following chapter, you will learn how to integrate all this information into a simple new plan that you can easily stick to. Get ready to eat well and feel great!

Walk
the
Weight
Away!

Nutrition Facts

Serving Size 1 oz. (2 cups 28g)
Servings Per Container about 1

Amount Per Serving

Calories 130	Calories from Fat 60
	% Daily Value*
Total Fat 6g	**10%**
Saturated Fat 1g	**5%**
Polyunsaturated Fat 1g	
Monounsaturated Fat 1g	
Cholesterol 0mg	**0%**
Sodium 150mg	**5%**
Total Carbohydrate 17g	**6%**
Dietary Fiber 2g	**8%**
Sugars 1g	
Protein 2g	
Vitamin A	0%
Vitamin C	0%
Calcium	0%
Iron	10%

* Percent Daily Values are based on a 2,000 calorie diet. Your Daily Values may be higher or lower depending on your calorie needs:

	Calories:	2,000	2,500
Total Fat	Less than	65g	80g
Sat Fat	Less than	20g	25g
Cholesterol	Less than	300mg	300mg
Sodium	Less than	2,400mg	2,400mg
Total Carbohydrate		300g	375g
Dietary Fiber		25g	30g

Ingredients: Corn Meal, Canola Oil, Aged Cheddar Cheese, (Milk, Salt, Cheese Cultures, Enzymes), Whey, Buttermilk, Maltodextrin, and Salt.

Reading a Food Label

• Note the order in which the ingredients are listed (those most abundant appear first).

• Read the nutrient information to determine the relative amounts of protein, carbs, fats, vitamins and minerals the food provides.

• Check the serving size and be aware that many packages contain two or three servings.

• Avoid foods that contain hydrogenated oils.

• Look for foods that strike a pyramid-based balance among carbohydrates, fats, and proteins.

Chapter 2
Losing Weight

The *Walk the Weight Away!* Nutrition Plan

What's so special about the *Walk the Weight Away!* nutrition plan? There's nothing trendy or earth-shattering to report, just sound nutrition advice. Our eating plan doesn't require you to purchase special supplements. Food choices aren't limited to pounds of assorted cabbage, and we don't require you to avoid a particular food group or nutrient. We don't promise results without effort and our program certainly is not revolutionary. On the contrary: Our principles are based on decades of tested and retested scientific research.

At the core of the *Walk the Weight Away!* nutrition plan are government recommendations based on the highest quality research to date.

Why are government recommendations more credible than most others? Motive is one reason. More than 50 percent of Americans over age 20 are overweight. The rate of diabetes is projected to double every 15 years. Healthcare costs, which the government has been trying desperately to contain, are soaring out of control. With these facts in mind, the government has an overwhelming reason to improve the health of our nation.

The quest for fame and fortune may be the driving force of other fitness promoters. "Lose 30 pounds in 30 days" sure makes a better headline than "Eat right and exercise more." Unfortunately, some research results are manipulated to benefit the pocketbooks of those funding the studies. The public is often misled because of a lack of expertise in the statistical skills needed to properly analyze these studies.

It Starts in the Kitchen

It's time to learn how to prepare your kitchen for weight loss victory. There are two primary goals:

1. Learn how to make healthy food choices.
2. Learn to identify appropriate portion sizes to meet your weight loss goals.

We're here to help, with suggestions about how to stock your pantry, cabinets, refrigerator, and freezer. Our easy-to-follow menus, delicious recipes, and expert hints and tips will help guide you to success.

Planning for Success

Let's face it, life is not always predictable and there will be times when you're not able to prepare the menu items we suggest. Plan ahead for those days by stocking your kitchen with quick-to-fix and grab-and-go foods. Some suggestions follow.

In the Refrigerator

- Condiments, including:
    catsup
    lemon juice
    lime juice
    mustard (several varieties)
    reduced-fat mayonnaise
    reduced-fat salad dressings
- Egg substitute
- Fresh fruit
- Fresh lemons and limes
- Lower fat luncheon meats including: turkey breast, chicken breast, and lean ham

- Fresh vegetables, including:
    - romaine or leaf lettuce
    - tomatoes
    - onions
    - green peppers
    - carrots
    - sweet potatoes
- Non-fat or 1 percent milk
- Non-fat or low fat yogurts
- Reduced-fat shredded and sliced cheeses
- String cheese

 ## Time-Saver Shortcut

Purchase ready-to-eat salad and pre-cut vegetables such as carrots, cauliflower, and broccoli. Store them in the refrigerator in a covered bowl partly filled with water and they'll stay fresh and crisp for several days.

In the Pantry

- Breakfast cereals that contain at least 2 grams of fiber per serving
- Canned beans
- Canned fruits in their own juice
- Canned vegetables
- Canned soups (low sodium)
- Canola and olive oils
- Dried fruits
- Instant hot cereals, including:
    - cream of wheat
    - grits
    - oatmeal
- Jams and jellies

- Individual servings of applesauce in a variety of flavors
- Microwave popcorn of the healthier variety
- Nuts packaged in individual servings (for portion control)
- Pancake mix (buckwheat, if you can find it)
- Pancake syrup
- Peanut butter (the freshly pressed varieties less saturated fat). Turn the container upside down after the first use then right side up after the next. This distributes the oil, making it easier to spread.
- Pizza sauce
- Prepared pasta sauces that are low in sodium
- Pretzels
- Quick-cooking white and brown rice
- Reduced-fat tuna lunch packs with crackers
- Tuna (packed in water)
- Vinegar (several varieties, including balsamic)

In the Freezer

- Frozen vegetables (several varieties)
- Chicken breast
- Frozen berries
- Frozen dinners of the healthier variety. Your maximum sodium intake should be 2400 milligrams per day, or a maximum of 800 milligrams per meal. Check for brands that meet these standards.
- Frozen fat-free chicken patties
- Frozen grilled fish fillets
- Frozen juice concentrates
- Frozen pancakes
- Frozen whole-grain waffles
- Veggie burgers
- Whole-grain breads (several varieties; bread freezes nicely and thaws quickly)
- Whole wheat pizza crust

Stock Up on Herbs and Spices

You know about salt and pepper, but are you neglecting the dozens of herbs and spices that can liven up the foods you eat? The table on page 37 offers ideas about which herbs and spices you might want to keep on hand and how to use them.

Low-Calorie, Low-Fat Cooking and Serving Methods

Cooking low-calorie, low-fat dishes doesn't take a long time, but your best intentions can be lost if you add butter or other fats at the table. It is important to learn how certain ingredients can add unwanted calories and fat to low-fat dishes. The following list provides examples of lower fat-cooking methods and tips on how to serve your low-fat dishes.

Low-Fat Cooking Methods

These cooking methods tend to be lower in fat:
- Baking
- Broiling
- Grilling
- Microwaving
- Roasting
- Sautéing (in cooking non- or low-fat cooking spray, small amounts of vegetable oil, or reduced sodium broth)
- Steaming
- Stir-frying

Walk
the
Weight
Away!

Herbs and Spices for Low-Fat, High-Flavor Cooking

Allspice	Beef, poultry, fruit, fish, ham, soups, stews
Basil	Beef, poultry, seafood, eggs, soups, stews, sauces, dips, salad dressings, vegetables, vinegar
Bay Leaf	Beef, fish, beans, soups, stews, potatoes, rice, vinegar, marinates, gravies
Cayenne Pepper	Beef, poultry, fish, soups, vegetables, pasta
Chili Powder	Chili, soups, vegetables, beans, salads
Chives	Soups, stews, sauces, dips, vegetables, salads, vinegars
Cilantro	Mexican and Asian dishes, curries, soups, stews, vegetables, fruit, desserts
Cinnamon	Pork, poultry, lamb, breads, vegetables, pasta, rice, fruit, desserts, coffee
Cloves	Beef, pork, lamb, soups, stews, vegetables, desserts
Cumin	Mexican, Indian, and Middle Eastern dishes; beef, lamb, pork, soups and stews; beans; chili; breads; sauces; dips; salad dressings; vinegar; desserts
Dill	Beef, poultry, seafood, vegetables, salads and salad dressing, marinates, dips, sauces, beans, breads, soups, vinegar
Garlic Powder	Beef, poultry, soups, stews, beans, vegetables, salads and salad dressings, marinades, sauces, dips, pasta, breads, rice
Ginger	Asian dishes, beef, poultry, fish, soups, stews, vegetables, breads, desserts
Ground Mustard	Beef, poultry, fish, potatoes, marinades, sauces, cheese dips, salads, salad dressing
Marjoram	Beef, poultry, seafood, soups, stews, sauces, dips, vegetables, breads, salads
Nutmeg	Beef, poultry, pork, soups, pasta, sauces. Vegetables, beans, fruit, desserts
Onion Powder	Beef, poultry, fish, soups, stews, beans, vegetables, breads, dips, sauces, marinades, salad dressings
Oregano	Beef, poultry, fish, pork, lamb, vegetables, sauces, salads, eggs, vinegar
Paprika	Beef, poultry, fish, soups, stews eggs, salads, salad dressing
Parsley	Beef, poultry, fish, soups, stews, salads, vegetables, eggs, pasta, cheese, breads, sauces, grains, vinegar
Rosemary	Beef, poultry, fish, lamb, vegetables, soups, stews, salads, potatoes, pasta, marinades, vinegar
Sage	Beef, poultry, pork, lamb, soups, stews, sauces, vegetables, pasta, casseroles, cheese, eggs, breads, grains, vinegar
Tarragon	Beef, poultry, fish, pasta, rice, grains, vegetables, marinades, vinegar
Thyme	Beef, poultry, fish, vegetables, soups, stews, salads, vinegar

Chapter 3

The *Walk the Weight Away!* Nutrition Plan

Reducing Calories and Fat

Eliminating some of the extra calories from your diet doesn't have to be a drag. All it takes is a little extra attention. The following examples offer ideas about how to reduce calories and fat when you prepare and serve food. You might be surprised at how easy it is.

- Two tablespoons of butter on a baked potato adds an extra 200 calories and 22 grams of fat. However, ¼ cup of salsa adds only 18 calories—and no fat!
- Two tablespoons of vinaigrette-style Italian salad dressing adds an extra 136 calories and 14 grams of fat. Reduced-fat Italian dressing adds only 30 calories and 2 grams of fat!

In fact, there are lots of low- and no-cal ways to liven up the foods you eat. Next time you want to add a little zip to the flavor of your meal, reach for one of these options:

- Catsup
- Fat-free or reduced-fat mayonnaise
- Fat-free or reduced-fat sour cream
- Fat-free or reduced-fat yogurt
- Ginger (fresh)
- Herbs: basil, cilantro, oregano, parsley, rosemary, sage, thyme
- Horseradish
- Jelly or fruit preserves (for English muffins, toast, or bagels)
- Lemon or lime juice
- Mustard
- Red pepper flakes
- Reduced-sodium soy sauce
- Reduced-fat or fat-free salad dressing
- Salsa
- Sodium-free salt substitute
- Spices: cinnamon, nutmeg, paprika, pepper
- Sprinkle of butter flavor (not made with real butter)
- Sprinkle of parmesan cheese (stronger flavor than most cheese)
- Vinegar

Walk
the
Weight
Away!

Alternatives to High-Fat / High-Calorie Foods

When you have a hankering for a high-fat, high-calorie treat, these low-calorie foods can provide you with healthy alternatives to your old favorites.

Dairy Products

INSTEAD OF	USE THESE LOWER-FAT ALTERNATIVES
Evaporated whole milk	Evaporated fat-free (skim), reduced-fat (2%) milk
Whole milk	Low-fat (1%) reduced-fat (2%), fat-free (skim) milk
Ice cream	Sorbet, sherbet, low-fat or fat-free frozen yogurt (check label for calorie content)
Whipping cream	Imitation whipped cream (made with fat-free [skim] milk), low-fat vanilla yogurt
Sour cream	Plain low-fat yogurt.
Cream cheese	Neufchâtel, "light" or fat-free cream cheese
Cheese	Reduced-calorie cheese, low-calorie processed cheeses
American cheese	Fat-free American cheese, other types of fat-free cheeses
Regular (4%) cottage cheese	Low-fat (1%) or reduced-fat (2%) cottage cheese
Whole milk mozzarella	Part-skim milk, low-moisture mozzarella cheese
Whole milk ricotta	Part-skim milk ricotta
Light cream (in coffee)	Half-and-half, nondairy creamer, low-fat (1%) or reduced-fat (2%) milk, non-fat dry milk powder

Cereals, Grains, and Pasta

INSTEAD OF	USE THESE LOWER-FAT ALTERNATIVES
Ramen noodles	Rice or noodles (spaghetti, macaroni.)
Pasta with Alfredo sauce	Pasta with marinara sauce
Pasta with cheese sauce	Pasta with vegetables (primavera)
Granola	Bran flakes, crispy rice; cooked grits or oatmeal; reduced-fat granola

Meat, Fish, and Poultry

INSTEAD OF	USE THESE LOWER-FAT ALTERNATIVES
Cold cuts or lunch meats (bologna, salami, liverwurst)	Low-fat cold cuts (95% to 97% fat-free lunch meats, low-fat pressed meats)
Hot dogs (regular)	Lower-fat or reduced calorie hot dogs
Bacon or sausage	Canadian bacon or lean ham
Regular ground beef	Extra lean ground beef such as ground round or ground turkey (read labels)
Chicken or turkey with skin; duck, or goose	Chicken or turkey without skin (white meat)
Oil-packed tuna	Water-packed tuna (rinse to reduce sodium content)
Beef (chuck, rib, brisket)	Beef—round, loin (trimmed of external fat/ choose select grades)
Pork (spareribs, untrimmed loin)	Pork tenderloin or trimmed, lean smoked ham
Frozen breaded fish or fried fish	Fish or shellfish, unbreaded (fresh, frozen, canned in water)
Whole eggs	Egg whites or egg substitute
Frozen TV dinners (High Fat)	Low-fat frozen TV dinners (less than 13 grams of fat per serving)
Chorizo sausage	Turkey sausage, drained well after cooking (read label); vegetarian sausage (made with tofu)

Baked Goods

INSTEAD OF	USE THESE LOWER-FAT ALTERNATIVES
Croissants or brioches	Hard French rolls or soft brown 'n serve rolls
Donuts, sweet rolls, muffins, scones, or pastries	English muffins, bagels, reduced-fat or fat-free muffins or scones.
Party crackers	Low-fat and low sodium crackers; saltine or soda crackers (choose varieties lower in sodium).
Cake (pound, chocolate, yellow)	Cake (angel food, white, gingerbread)
Cookies	Reduced-fat or fat-free cookies (graham crackers, ginger snaps, fig bars)

Snacks and Sweets

INSTEAD OF	USE THESE LOWER-FAT ALTERNATIVES
Nuts	Popcorn (air-popped or light microwave), fruits, vegetables
Ice cream	Frozen yogurt, frozen fruit or chocolate pudding bars
Custards or puddings (made with whole milk)	Puddings (made with skim milk)

Fats, Oils, and Salad Dressings

INSTEAD OF	USE THESE LOWER-FAT ALTERNATIVES
Regular margarine or butter	Light spread margarines, diet margarine, or whipped butter
Regular mayonnaise	Light or diet mayonnaise or mustard
Regular salad dressings	Reduced-calorie fat-free salad dressings; lemon juice; plain or herb flavored; wine vinegar
Butter or margarine on toast or bread	Jelly, jam, or honey on bread or toast

Chapter 3

The *Walk the Weight Away!* Nutrition Plan

Oils, shortening, or lard   Nonstick cooking spray for stir-frying or sautéing

Note: You can substitute applesauce or prune puree for up to one-third the fat (butter, oil) called for in a baking recipe.

Miscellaneous

INSTEAD OF	USE THESE LOWER-FAT ALTERNATIVES
Canned cream soups	Canned broth-based soups
Canned beans and franks	Canned baked beans in tomato sauce
Gravy (homemade with fat and/or milk)	Gravy mixes made with water or homemade with the fat skimmed off using fat-free milk
Fudge sauce	Chocolate syrup
Avocado on sandwiches	Cucumber slices or lettuce leaves
Guacamole dip or refried beans with lard	Salsa

Walk the Weight Away! Meal Plans

Look through the workbook section that begins on page 152 and you'll notice that on each day we offer three menus—breakfast, lunch, dinner—and one snack. (You'll find recipes for bulleted menu items listed in the next section.)

Our meal plans are designed in accordance with the Dietary Guidelines for Americans and the Food Guide Pyramid. Each meal is packed with nutrient-dense foods (foods abundant in vitamins, minerals, and additional nutrients needed for good health compared with the calories they contain).

Here's the breakdown:

- Each daily menu is designed to provide about 1,600 calories.
- Each meal is roughly 400 calories; snacks range from 50 to 150 calories.
- Proteins comprise 12 to 20 percent of total calories.
- Carbohydrates comprise 55 to 60 percent of daily calories.
- Fats comprise 25 to 30 percent of daily calories.

And of course, when selecting recipes and planning menus, we kept good nutrition in mind.

We also considered the ease in acquiring ingredients and the popularity of menu items. Every daily menu may not provide 100 percent of the recommended amount of every single nutrient. Some days will contain a little more; some days, a little less. However, over the course of a few days, you can be sure that your nutrient intake will balance out and all of your needs will be met.

Now, if you've ever visited a fast food restaurant (and we all have), you've mastered the value meal system. If you want to choose the Number Two meal every time you drive up, you can. This is how the *Walk the Weight Away!* meal plan works. If a particular menu item doesn't appeal to you, just substitute another "value" meal (just don't super-size it).

For instance, for breakfast on day two of Phase II, we recommend a breakfast of 1 Graham Cracker Muffin, 1 cup non-fat milk, and 1 small banana. If that breakfast doesn't appeal to you, just choose a breakfast from another day—maybe you prefer the Potato & Cheese Omelet, 1 slice of whole wheat toast with 1 teaspoon of butter, and a wedge of cantaloupe from another week. That's fine—it's entirely up to you. Having this freedom to vary menu choices ensures that you eat a diet that (1) appeals to your personal taste and (2) contains adequate amounts of the nutrients required for optimal energy and health. Don't be afraid to experiment with a number of these easy-to-prepare meals, just let your taste buds navigate.

When reviewing your menus, you may want to plan a few days' worth at a time. This planning will allow you to use up ingredients you already have. For example, leftover chicken from tonight's dinner can be used in chicken salad for tomorrow's lunch. Some of the vegetables for tomorrow's dinner can be eaten raw at lunch today. This makes grocery shopping less cumbersome and keeps your refrigerator from becoming a science project.

Date:

Nutrition Guide

Suggested Menu

Breakfast

3 Whole Wheat Pancakes with Strawberry Syrup

1 cup non-fat milk

Lunch

Heart-Healthy Egg Salad Sandwich

raw cucumber slices

1 apple

Dinner

1 portion Southwestern Pork Tenderloin

1 ear corn

½ plate mixed vegetable salad

1 tablespoon low-fat salad dressing

Snacks

1 cup juice

Are you a life-long member of the clean plate club? Maybe it's time to give up your membership. Finishing everything on your plate just because it's there isn't necessarily a healthy way to eat. In restaurants, where portions tend to be gargantuan, you may decide to eat only half the food and save the other half for the following day's lunch. And at home, serve yourself small portions that you know you can finish without feeling stuffed.

Breakfast   time: 7:30 a.m.

What I ate _cereal, orange juice_

What I was doing while I ate _making a shopping list_

Hunger level _a little hungry_

Lunch   time: 2:00 p.m.

What I ate _hamburger with lettuce & tomato_

What I was doing while I ate _reading the paper_

Hunger level _very hungry_

Dinner   time: 7:30 p.m.

What I ate _ravioli & grilled chicken, red wine._

What I was doing while I ate _on a date_

Hunger level _very hungry_

Snack   time: 4:00 p.m.

What I ate _ice-cream_

What I was doing while I ate _watching tv_

Hunger level _not hungry_

Water ✓✓✓✓✓✓✓

Remember to drink 8 glasses of water

I feel __ about how I ate today:

☐ satisfied
☐ proud
☐ disappointed
☑ other _okay_

My goal for tomorrow _Not to eat when I'm not hungry._

About Our Recipe Analyses

All of the *Walk the Weight Away!* recipes are analyzed for total calories, fat, saturated fat, protein, carbohydrates (carb), fiber, cholesterol (chol), and sodium. In those analyses, we abbreviate grams as "g" and milligrams as "mg." We use Food Processor software (by ESHA Research), version 8.0, for recipe analysis.

Walk the **Weight Away!**

The *Walk the Weight Away!* Recipes

Chapter 3

The *Walk the Weight Away!* Nutrition Plan

Blueberry Muffins

Makes 12 muffins

Ingredients

2 cups all-purpose flour

⅓ cup granulated sugar

1 teaspoon baking powder

1 teaspoon baking soda

¼ cup orange juice

2 tablespoons canola oil

1 teaspoon vanilla extract

1 8-ounce container vanilla or blueberry yogurt

1 large egg

1 cup blueberries (frozen can be used if thawed)

Directions

1 Preheat oven to 400°F. In a large bowl, combine the flour, sugar, baking powder, and baking soda.

2 In a small bowl, combine the juice, oil, vanilla, yogurt, egg, and blueberries.

3 Spoon batter into a lined muffin tin. Bake 17 to 19 minutes, until a toothpick inserted in the center of each muffin comes out clean.

Calories 154 (19% from fat); Fat 3g (sat 0g); Protein 4g; Carb 28g; Fiber 1g; Chol 19mg; Sodium 165mg

Walk the **Weight** Away!

Brunch Wraps

Serves 4

Ingredients

1 package (10-ounces) frozen, chopped spinach, thawed and
drained

½ cup non-fat sour cream

2 teaspoons Italian seasoning

4 large flour tortillas

2 cups chopped salad mix

1 cup chopped tomatoes

1 cup cooked, diced chicken

¼ cup chopped scallions

¼ cup shredded low-fat mozzarella cheese

Directions

1. In a small bowl, combine the spinach, sour cream, and Italian seasoning. Mix well.

2. Spread ¼ cup of the mixture onto each tortilla, covering it completely. Divide the salad mix, tomatoes, chicken, scallions, and cheese evenly among the tortillas.

3. Fold the tortilla top and bottom over the filling, then roll to form a tightly rolled sandwich.

4. Wrap each roll in plastic wrap and refrigerate at least 2 hours. Serve chilled.

Calories 286 (23% from fat); Fat 7g (sat 2g); Protein 19g; Carb 37g; Fiber 3g; Chol 31mg; Sodium 687mg

Cheesy Potato Omelette

Serves 2

Ingredients

1 large egg

¾ cup egg substitute

2 teaspoons unsalted butter

¾ cup diced cooked warm potatoes

¾ cup low-fat cheese

Directions

1. In a small bowl, mix egg and egg substitute.

2. In a medium skillet set over medium heat, melt the butter. Add the eggs and cook until not quite set.

3. Spoon potatoes and cheese onto omelette. Cover and cook until eggs are completely set.

4. Fold omelette and serve.

Calories 257 (39% from fat); Fat 11g (sat 6g); Protein 24g; Carb 14g; Fiber 1g; Chol 130mg; Sodium 183mg

Walk
the
Weight
Away!

French Toast

Serves 4

Ingredients

½ carton egg substitute

1 large egg

2 tablespoons nonfat milk

½ teaspoon vanilla extract

¼ teaspoon ground cinnamon

8 slices whole-grain bread

Directions

1 In a shallow dish, whisk together the egg substitute, egg, milk, vanilla, and cinnamon.

2 Coat a skillet with non-stick cooking spray. Heat over medium heat.

3 Working in batches, soak bread in egg mixture, letting excess drip off. Transfer bread to skillet and fry until browned, turning once.

Calories 184 (16% from fat); Fat 3g (sat 1g); Protein 13g; Carb 26g; Fiber 3g; Chol 53mg; Sodium 355mg

Breakfast

Chapter 3
The *Walk the Weight Away!* Nutrition Plan

Graham Cracker Muffins

Makes 8 muffins

Ingredients

3 cups crushed graham crackers

¼ cup granulated sugar

2 teaspoons baking powder

1 cup nonfat milk

¼ cup egg substitute

1 tablespoon vanilla extract

Directions

1. Preheat oven to 400°F. Line a muffin tin with cups.

2. In a large bowl, combine the graham crackers, sugar, and baking powder.

3. Add the milk, egg substitute, and vanilla to the dry ingredients. Stir until just blended.

4. Spoon batter into muffin tin. Bake 14 to 16 minutes, until a toothpick inserted into the center of each muffin comes out clean.

Calories 187 (20% from fat); Fat 4g (sat 1g); Protein 4g; Carb 33g; Fiber 1g; Chol 1mg; Sodium 346mg

Greek Omelette

Serves 2

Ingredients

1 large egg

¾ cup egg substitute

½ cup cooked, warm, chopped spinach

¼ cup finely chopped, cooked onion

1 ounce crumbled feta cheese

Directions

1. In a small bowl mix the egg and egg substitute.

2. Spray an omelette pan or skillet with non-stick cooking spray. Set over medium heat.

3. Pour the egg mixture into the skillet. Cover and cook for 1 to 2 minutes, or until eggs are nearly set. Spoon the spinach, onion, and cheese onto the eggs. Cover and cook for 30 seconds more.

4. Fold over omelette and serve.

Calories 147 (37% from fat); Fat 6g (sat 3g); Protein 16g; Carb 7g; Fiber 2g; Chol 116mg; Sodium 397mg

Breakfast

Chapter 3

The *Walk the Weight Away!* Nutrition Plan

Strawberry Orange Muffins

Makes 12 muffins

Ingredients

1 cup chopped strawberries

⅓ cup granulated sugar

⅔ cup plus 1 tablespoon orange juice, divided

1 ½ cups whole wheat flour

½ cup soy flour

2 teaspoons baking powder

1 teaspoon baking soda

½ teaspoon nutmeg

2 tablespoons canola oil

2 egg whites, lightly beaten

1 ½ teaspoons freshly grated orange peel

Directions

1. Preheat oven to 350°F.

2. In a medium bowl, combine the strawberries, sugar, and 1 tablespoon of orange juice. Set aside.

3. In a large bowl, combine the flours, baking powder, baking soda, and nutmeg.

4. In a small bowl, whisk together the remaining orange juice, oil, and egg whites.

5. Add the egg white mixture to the dry ingredients. Mix until blended. Add the strawberry mixture and orange peel.

6. Pour the batter into non-stick muffin cups. Bake for 15 minutes or until a toothpick inserted in the muffin centers comes out clean.

Calories (25% from fat) 124; Fat 3g (sat 0g); Protein 4g; Carb 21g; Fiber 3g; Chol 0mg; Sodium 197mg

Strawberry Syrup

Makes ¾ cup

Ingredients

½ cup pure maple syrup

½ cup sliced strawberries (if frozen, thawed)

Directions

1. Combine syrup and berries in a microwave safe dish. Cover with plastic wrap.

2. Microwave on HIGH until mixture begins to boil.

3. Let stand for 1 minute and serve.

Calories 444 (1% from fat); Fat 1g (sat 0g); Protein 1g; Carb 113g; Fiber 2g; Chol 0mg; Sodium 15mg

Chapter 3
The *Walk the Weight Away!* Nutrition Plan

Whole Wheat Pancakes

Serves 8

Ingredients

1 cup whole wheat flour

½ teaspoon baking soda

½ teaspoon baking powder

1 ½ teaspoons granulated sugar

¼ cup egg substitute

1 cup non-fat milk

1 tablespoon canola oil

¼ teaspoon vanilla

Directions

1. In a large bowl, combine the flour, baking soda, baking powder, and sugar.

2. In a small bowl, combine the egg substitute, milk, oil, and vanilla. Whisk well.

3. Working in batches, spray a large skillet with non-stick cooking spray. Heat over medium-high heat. Add batter by ⅓ cupfuls; when pancake looks bubbly on top and around the edges, flip and cook for 1 minute more.

Calories 94 (28% from fat); Fat 3g (sat 0g); Protein 4g; Carb 14g; Fiber 2g; Chol 1mg; Sodium 143mg

Chicken Salad Sandwiches Italiano

Makes 2 Sandwiches

Ingredients

1 chicken breast, cooked and chopped

¼ teaspoon Italian seasoning

1 celery stalk, chopped fine

1 scallion, chopped fine

1 tablespoon lemon juice

¼ cup low-fat mayonnaise

5 seedless grapes, each cut into 4 pieces

lettuce and tomato slices

4 slices whole grain bread, toasted

Directions

1. In a small bowl combine chicken, Italian seasoning, celery, and scallion. Mix well.

2. Add the lemon juice, mayonnaise, and grapes; mix well.

3. Serve salad, topped with lettuce and tomato, between 2 slices of toasted whole grain bread.

Calories 301 (14% from fat); Fat 5g (sat 1g); Protein 23g; Carb 45g; Fiber 8g; Chol 40mg; Sodium 589mg

Lunch

55

Chapter 3
The *Walk the Weight Away!* Nutrition Plan

Lunch

Heart-Healthy Egg Salad Sandwiches

Makes 2 Sandwiches

Ingredients

½ cup egg substitute

3 hard-cooked egg whites

¼ cup low-fat mayonnaise

1 tablespoon Dijon mustard

2 chopped scallions

2 chopped celery stalks

¼ teaspoon Tabasco sauce

lettuce and tomato slices

4 slices whole-grain bread, toasted

Directions

1 Coat a medium skillet with non-stick cooking spray. Add egg substitute and cook, covered, over low heat (do not scramble) until cooked through. Transfer to cutting board.

2 Chop cooked egg substitute and egg whites; transfer to a medium bowl.

3 Add mayonnaise, Dijon, scallions, celery, and Tabasco to eggs; mix well.

4 Serve salad, topped with lettuce and tomato, on toast.

Calories 293 (12% from fat); Fat 4g (sat 1g); Protein 21g; Carb 47g; Fiber 9g; Chol 3mg; Sodium 939mg

56

Walk the **Weight** **Away!**

Lemon Hummus Sandwiches

Serves 4

Ingredients

1 can (15-ounces) garbanzo beans, rinsed and drained

½ cup nonfat, plain yogurt

1 tablespoon lemon pepper seasoning

¼ cup shredded carrots

3 tablespoons chopped scallions

1 large romaine lettuce leaf

4 whole wheat pita bread halves

Directions

1. In a blender pitcher, combine the beans, yogurt, lemon pepper seasoning, and ¼ cup water. Puree until smooth; transfer mixture to a small bowl.

2. Stir carrots and scallions into the chickpea mixture.

3. Line the inside of each pita half with lettuce; add one-quarter of the chickpea mixture.

Calories 206 (8% from fat); Fat 2g (sat 0g); Protein 9g; Carb 40g; Fiber 7g; Chol 1mg; Sodium 804mg

Lunch

57

Updated Sloppy Joe Sandwiches

Serves 6

Ingredients

1 cup dry textured soy protein (TVP)

¼ cup plus 1 tablespoon bottled chili sauce

1 cup chopped onion

½ cup finely chopped zucchini

½ cup chopped bell pepper

8-ounce can tomato sauce

½ teaspoon chili powder

2 teaspoons Worcestershire sauce

1 teaspoon vinegar

6 hamburger buns

Directions

1 Place the TVP in a medium bowl.

2 In a small bowl, combine 1 tablespoon of the chili sauce and 1 cup boiling water. Pour mixture over the TVP to rehydrate it.

3 In a medium skillet, sauté the onion, zucchini, and pepper in a little water until tender.

4 Add the soy mixture, tomato sauce, remaining chili sauce, chili powder, Worcestershire, and vinegar to the vegetable mixture. Simmer 5 minutes.

5 Serve on the hamburger buns.

Calories 270 (11% from fat); Fat 3g (sat 0g); Protein 26g; Carb 43g; Fiber 11g; Chol 0mg; Sodium 881mg

Lunch

Walk the **Weight** Away!

Veggie Pita Sandwiches

Serves 2

Ingredients

¼ cup plain yogurt

1 teaspoon lemon juice

2 tablespoons low-fat Italian dressing

¼ cucumber, thinly sliced

⅛ cup shredded carrots

⅛ cup alfalfa sprouts

2 slices tomato, chopped

2 tablespoons black olive slices

1 whole wheat pita cut into two pockets

Directions

1 In a medium bowl, combine the yogurt, lemon juice, and salad dressing. Stir in the cucumber, carrots, sprouts, tomato, and olive slices.

2 Stuff into pita pockets; serve.

Calories 122 (25% from fat); Fat 3g (sat 0g); Protein 4g; Carb 21g; Fiber 3g; Chol 1mg; Sodium 467mg

Dinner

59

Baked Chicken Siciliano

Serves 8

Ingredients

1 15-ounce can tomato sauce

4 teaspoons Italian seasoning, divided

½ cup grated Parmesan cheese, plus extra for sprinkling

8 boneless, skinless chicken breasts

Directions

1 Preheat oven to 400°F.

2 In a medium bowl, combine tomato sauce, 3 teaspoons of the Italian seasoning, and ½ cup of the Parmesan.

3 Coat chicken with mixture. Place chicken in baking dish and sprinkle with remaining Parmesan and Italian seasoning.

4 Bake for 40 minutes or until chicken juices run clear when pierced with a knife.

Calories 182 (19% from fat); Fat 4g (sat 2g); Protein 31g; Carb 5g; Fiber 1g; Chol 74mg; Sodium 538mg

Dinner

Walk
the
Weight
Away!

Barbecued Pork

Serves 4

Ingredients

1 ¼ pounds boneless pork shoulder

1 onion, diced

2 tablespoons minced garlic

2 tablespoons granulated sugar

½ teaspoon Dijon mustard

1 cup catsup

3 tablespoons Worcestershire sauce

Directions

1 Cut pork crosswise into ¼-inch slices.

2 In a small bowl, combine onion, garlic, sugar, mustard, catsup, and Worcestershire. Mix well.

3 Place pork and sauce into a slow cooker. Cook on low for 6 hours, or until pork is tender.

Calories 324 (24% from fat); Fat 9g (sat 3g); Protein 32g; Carb 29g; Fiber 2g; Chol 97mg; Sodium 920mg

Dinner

Chapter 3
The *Walk the Weight Away!* Nutrition Plan

Dinner

Buttery Almond Fish

Serves 2

Ingredients

1 ½ tablespoons dried butter substitute

1 ½ teaspoons lemon pepper seasoning

½ teaspoon lime juice

½ teaspoon honey

8 ounces boneless whitefish fillets

1 ½ tablespoons sliced toasted almonds

Directions

1 Preheat broiler. In a small bowl combine the butter substitute, lemon pepper seasoning, lime juice, honey, and ½ teaspoon water. Mix well.

2 Broil the fish 6 to 8 inches from the heat for 5 minutes, turning once.

3 Spread mixture on fish; broil another 4 to 5 minutes.

4 Sprinkle with almonds and serve.

Calories 141 (20% from fat); Fat 3g (sat 0g); Protein 21g; Carb 6g; Fiber 1g; Chol 49mg; Sodium 452mg

Walk the **Weight Away!**

Cheese Ravioli Soup

Serves 6

Ingredients

4 20-ounce cans low-sodium, low-fat chicken broth

1 16-ounce package frozen red pepper stir-fry

4 tablespoons Italian seasoning

1 13-ounce package frozen mini cheese ravioli

Directions

1 In a medium saucepan, combine the broth, stir-fry mix, and Italian seasoning.

2 Bring mixture to a boil; add ravioli. Reduce heat and simmer for 10 to 15 minutes.

Calories 238 (27% from fat); Fat 7g (sat 4g); Protein 17g; Carb 31g; Fiber 4g; Chol 31mg; Sodium 764mg

Oaty Beef Burgers

Serves 6

Ingredients

½ pound extra lean hamburger

1 ½ cups uncooked oatmeal

½ small onion, chopped

1 cup marinara sauce

6 hamburger rolls

Directions

1 In a medium bowl, combine the hamburger, oatmeal, onion, and marinara sauce. Mix well.

2 Shape mixture into 6 hamburger patties. Cook until burgers and serve on rolls.

Calories 256 (26% from fat); Fat 7g (sat 3g); Protein 15g; Carb 33g; Fiber 2g; Chol 14mg; Sodium 430mg

Chapter 3

The *Walk the Weight Away!* Nutrition Plan

Chicken and Sun-Dried Tomato Pasta Salad

Serves 6

Ingredients

2 cups uncooked bow-tie pasta

1 14-ounce can artichoke hearts, drained and chopped

1 ½ cups chopped, cooked chicken

2 cups cooked broccoli florets

½ cup sun-dried tomato strips in oil

2 tablespoons balsamic vinegar

4 teaspoons Italian seasoning

Directions

1. Prepare pasta according to package directions. Drain and place in a large bowl.

2. Stir in remaining ingredients. Serve chilled.

Calories 432 (18% from fat); Fat 8g (sat 1g); Protein 24g; Carb 70g; Fiber 7g; Chol 26mg; Sodium 318mg

Dinner

Walk
the
Weight
Away!

Chicken Cacciatore

Serves 6

Ingredients

2 teaspoons olive oil

6 boneless, skinless chicken breasts

¾ cup chopped green bell pepper

¾ cup sliced mushrooms

1 14 ½-ounce can pasta-ready tomatoes, undrained

2 tablespoons parsley

1 ½ tablespoons Italian seasoning

Directions

1 Heat olive oil in large skillet over medium heat. Add chicken and sauté until browned on both sides.

2 Add the pepper, mushrooms, tomatoes, parsley, and Italian seasoning to chicken. Simmer, uncovered, for 10 to 12 minutes, or until juices run clear when the chicken is pierced with a knife.

Calories 190 (23% from fat); Fat 5g (sat 1g); Protein 28g; Carb 8g; Fiber 2g; Chol 73mg; Sodium 338mg

Dinner

65

Dinner

Chicken Del Jardin

Serves 4

Ingredients

4 boneless, skinless chicken breasts

½ teaspoon chili powder

½ teaspoon garlic powder

½ teaspoon thyme

½ teaspoon onion powder

4 small zucchini, halved and cut into ¼-inch-thick slices

1 8-ounce can no-salt-added corn

⅔ cup mild picante sauce

Directions

1 Coat a large skillet with non-stick cooking spray. Pound chicken breasts to a ¼-inch thickness.

2 Set skillet over medium heat. Add chicken to hot skillet and cook for 2 minutes. In a small bowl, combine chili powder, garlic powder, thyme, and onion powder.

3 Turn the chicken and sprinkle cooked side with the spice mixture. Cook for 1 minute more, until thoroughly cooked.

4 Transfer chicken to a serving platter and cover with foil.

5 Add zucchini, corn, and picante to skillet. Cook over medium-low heat until zucchini is tender.

6 Top chicken with zucchini mixture and serve.

Calories 221 (16% from fat); Fat 4g (sat 1g); Protein 30g; Carb 17g; Fiber 3g; Chol 73mg; Sodium 601mg

Walk the **Weight Away!**

Chunky Beef and Vegetable Soup

Serves 8

Ingredients

1 tablespoon canola oil

1 ¼ pounds beef shank crosscuts

1 cup diced celery

½ cup chopped onion

1 10-ounce package frozen mixed vegetables

1 cup salt-free canned tomatoes, chopped

1 6-ounce can salt-free tomato paste

1 tablespoon granulated sugar

2 teaspoons garlic powder

2 teaspoons vinegar

2 tablespoons cornstarch

Directions

1 Heat oil in a large saucepan set over medium heat. Add beef and sauté until browned on all sides.

2 Add celery, onion, and 2 quarts water to the pot. Bring to a boil, reduce heat, and simmer for 2 hours. Remove beef from saucepan and let cool.

3 Add the vegetables, tomatoes, tomato paste, sugar, garlic powder, and vinegar to the soup. Stir well and simmer for 1 hour. Meanwhile, remove beef from shanks and cut into small cubes.

4 Return cubed meat to the soup. In a small bowl, combine the cornstarch with ½ cup cold water. Mix until smooth. Add to the soup and stir until thickened slightly.

Calories 162 (34% from fat); Fat 6g (sat 2g); Protein 11g; Carb 17g; Fiber 3g; Chol 22mg; Sodium 141mg

Dinner

67

Citrus Orange Roughy

Serves 4

Ingredients

1 pound orange roughy or catfish fillets

1 teaspoon dried basil

1 teaspoon garlic powder

2 slices fresh orange

2 slices fresh lemon

2 slices fresh lime

Directions

1 Preheat oven to 350°F. Arrange fish in baking dish.

2 Spring fish with basil and garlic powder. Top with fruit slices.

3 Bake 15 to 20 minutes, until fish is opaque and easily flakes with fork.

Calories 131 (8% from fat); Fat 1g (sat 0g); Protein 22g; Carb 8g; Fiber 2g; Chol 29mg; Sodium 93mg

Walk the **Weight** Away!

Crispy Chicken

Serves 4

Ingredients

1 ½ cups crushed unsweetened bran cereal

1 ½ teaspoon minced garlic

1 ½ teaspoon paprika

1 tablespoon canola or olive oil

¼ cup nonfat milk

4 boneless, skinless chicken breasts

Directions

1 Preheat oven to 350°F.

2 In shallow dish combine the cereal, garlic, and paprika.

3 In another shallow dish, whisk the oil into the milk.

4 Dunk the chicken into the milk and then into the cereal mixture, coating well, but letting excess drop off.

5 Arrange chicken in baking dish and bake 18 minutes. Turn and continue baking 10 minutes more, or until juices run clear when chicken is pierced with a knife.

Calories 131 (8% from fat); Fat 1g (sat 0g); Protein 22g; Carb 8g; Fiber 2g; Chol 29mg; Sodium 93mg

Dinner

69

Grilled Marinated Salmon

Serves 4

Ingredients

¼ cup light soy sauce

½ cup sweet wine

2 tablespoons lime juice

4 salmon fillets (about 4 ounces each)

3 tablespoons chopped scallions

Directions

1 In a shallow dish, combine the soy sauce, wine, and lime juice.

2 Add salmon to the marinade. Cover and refrigerate at least 2 hours.

3 Preheat grill pan or counter. Grill fish for 2 minutes. Turn and continue grilling for 1 minute more.

4 Sprinkle with scallions and serve.

Calories 233 (32% from fat); Fat 8g (sat 1g); Protein 26g; Carb 5g; Fiber 0g; Chol 72mg; Sodium 960mg

Kielbasa Kebabs

Serves 6

Ingredients

1 medium zucchini, cut into 1-inch chunks

1 medium onion, cut into 1-inch chunks

1 medium red bell pepper, cored and cut into 1-inch chunks

1 cup reduced-fat Italian salad dressing

1 pound turkey kielbasa cut into 1-inch chunks

6 wooden skewers

Directions

1 In a medium bowl, combine the zucchini, onion, pepper, and salad dressing. Cover and refrigerate at least 2 hours.

2 Just before grilling, soak skewers in water for 30 minutes. Preheat grill.

3 Remove vegetables from marinade; discard excess. Thread kielbasa and vegetables on skewer, alternating ingredients.

5 Grill about 8 minutes, until vegetables are tender and kielbasa is cooked through.

6 Serve with rice.

Calories 155 (38% from fat); Fat 6g (sat 2g); Protein 13g; Carb 11g; Fiber 2g; Chol 51mg; Sodium 1242mg

Dinner

71

Pasta Primavera

Serves 8

Ingredients

1 16-ounce package angel hair pasta

2 tablespoons olive oil

2 tablespoons minced garlic

½ cup chopped onion

1 cup thin-sliced zucchini slices

4 tomatoes, chopped

1 cup mushroom slices

2 tablespoons grated Parmesan cheese

Directions

1 Cook pasta according to package directions.

2 Meanwhile, in a medium skillet set over medium heat, sauté garlic and onion in olive oil for 1 minute.

2 Add zucchini and sauté 1 minute.

3 Add tomatoes and mushrooms; sauce until heated through.

4 Drain pasta and transfer to serving platter or bowl. Top with vegetable mixture, sprinkle with cheese, and serve.

Calories 275 (16% from fat); Fat 5g (sat 1g); Protein 9g; Carb 49g; Fiber 3g; Chol 1mg; Sodium 117mg

Pizza Primavera

Serves 8

Ingredients

1 12-inch ready-to-use thick-crust pizza crust

5 ounces pizza sauce

½ cup chopped mushrooms

½ cup sliced bell pepper

½ cup chopped fresh broccoli

½ cup chopped scallions

½ cup low-fat, grated mozzarella cheese

¼ cup grated Parmesan cheese

Directions

1. Preheat oven to 450°F. Place crust on a cookie sheet

2. Spread sauce on crust; sprinkle on mushrooms, pepper, broccoli, and scallions. Top with cheese.

3. Bake for 7 to 9 minutes. Cool slightly, cut into 8 wedges, and serve.

Calories 138 (21% from fat); Fat 3g (sat 1g); Protein 7g; Carb 20g; Fiber 1g; Chol 6mg; Sodium 369mg

Chapter 3

The *Walk the Weight Away!* Nutrition Plan

Pork Chops Dijon

Serves 2

Ingredients

1 teaspoon low-sodium chicken broth

2 tablespoons honey

4 teaspoons Dijon mustard

1 teaspoon garlic powder

1 teaspoon Italian seasoning

2 pork loin chops

Directions

1 Preheat oven to 350°F.

2 In a baking dish, combine the broth, honey, mustard, garlic powder, and seasoning.

3 Arrange chops in the baking dish. Bake, covered, for 25 minutes. Uncover and cook 10 minutes more.

Calories 224 (30% from fat); Fat 8g (sat 2g); Protein 20g; Carb 20g; Fiber 0g; Chol 49mg; Sodium 460mg

Note: Freeze leftover broth in ice cube trays. Once frozen, transfer the cubes to a plastic bag and use them to flavor soups and vegetables.

Pork Tenderloin in Cream Sauce

Serves 6

Ingredients

1   pork tenderloin (about 1 ½ pounds)

1 teaspoon black pepper

2 10 ¾-ounce cans condensed reduced-fat cream of mushroom soup

1 can sliced mushrooms, drained

Directions

1 Place tenderloin in a slow cooker; sprinkle with pepper.

2 Pour soup and mushrooms over tenderloin.

3 Cover and cook on low for 8 hours.

*Calories 170 (28% from fat); Fat 5g (sat 2g); Protein 24g; Carb 6g; Fiber 1g;
    Chol 65mg; Sodium 546mg*

Dinner

75

Dinner

Pot Roast and Vegetables

Serves 8

Ingredients

6 small potatoes, peeled and quartered

1 small bag baby carrots

1 large onion, peeled and sliced

1 beef sirloin pot roast (about 3 pounds)

2 tablespoons minced garlic

1 teaspoon pepper

1 teaspoon paprika

¼ cup Worcestershire sauce

1 can low-sodium beef broth

1 bay leaf

Directions

1. Place the potatoes, carrots, and onion in a slow cooker.

2. Rub meat with garlic, pepper, and paprika; place on top of vegetables.

3. In a small bowl combine the Worcestershire and broth; pour over the beef.

4. Place bay leaf on top of vegetables.

5. Cook on low for about 8 hours.

Calories 547 (38% from fat); Fat 23g (sat 9g); Protein 51g; Carb 32g; Fiber 5g; Chol 139mg; Sodium 236mg

Walk the **Weight** Away!

Southwestern Pork Tenderloin

Serves 6

Ingredients

2 tablespoons chili powder

1 ½ teaspoons oregano

¾ teaspoon cumin

2 tablespoons minced garlic

1 tablespoon vegetable oil

1 pork tenderloin (about 1 ½ pounds); split in half lengthwise

Directions

1 In a small bowl, combine the chili powder, oregano, cumin, garlic, and vegetable.

2 Rub the mixture over entire tenderloin. Cover and refrigerate at least 2 hours.

3 Preheat grill. Grill tenderloin 15 minutes, or until thermometer inserted in the middle reads 160°F.

Calories 156 (32% from fat); Fat 6g (sat 2g); Protein 23g; Carb 3g; Fiber 1g; Chol 63mg; Sodium 72mg

Dinner

Chapter 3

The *Walk the Weight Away!* Nutrition Plan

Spaghetti Squash Pomodoro

Serves 4

Ingredients

1 spaghetti squash (about 3 pounds)

1 tablespoon olive oil

2 cups ripe tomatoes, chopped

½ cup grated Romano cheese

1 tablespoon Italian seasoning

¼ cup toasted almonds

Directions

1 Preheat oven to 350°F.

2 Pierce the squash in 3 places with a knife. Bake until squash can be easily depressed with a finger. Immediately cut in half and cool 10 minutes. Scoop out seeds; discard.

3 Meanwhile, combine the olive oil, tomatoes, cheese, and Italian seasoning in a large bowl.

4 Comb strands out of squash with a fork until only the shell remains.

5 Add squash to sauce; mix well.

6 Top with nuts and serve.

Calories 159 (33% from fat); Fat 6g (sat 2g); Protein 6g; Carb 24g; Fiber 5g; Chol 5mg; Sodium 330mg

Walk the **Weight** Away!

Spunky Vegetarian Chili

Serves 6

Ingredients

2 15 ounce-cans red kidney beans, rinsed and drained

2 14 ½-ounce cans chunky, chili style tomatoes, undrained

1 cup chopped onion

1 cup chopped green bell pepper

1 tablespoon chili powder

1 teaspoon ground cumin

½ cup low-fat shredded Cheddar cheese

Directions

1. In a large pot, combine beans, tomatoes, onion, pepper, chili powder, and cumin. Simmer covered for 20 minutes, stirring occasionally.

2. Spoon chili into bowls; garnish with Cheddar and serve.

Calories 241 (6% from fat); Fat 2g (sat 0g); Protein 15g; Carb 45g; Fiber 16g; Chol 2mg; Sodium 735mg

Dinner

79

Chapter 3
The *Walk the Weight Away!* Nutrition Plan

Stovetop Lentil Casserole

Serves 6

Ingredients

2 cans lentil soup

1 medium carrot, diced

2 teaspoons Italian seasoning

1 cup chunky tomato sauce

3 ounces smoked turkey sausage

2 scallions, chopped

Directions

1. In a medium saucepan, combine the soup, carrot, and Italian seasoning. Bring mixture to a boil, reduce heat and simmer, stirring often.

2. Mash lentils in soup with a potato masher; add tomato sauce and sausage.

3. Simmer 10 minutes, garnish with scallions, and serve.

Calories 97 (18% from fat); Fat 2g (sat 1g); Protein 6g; Carb 14g; Fiber 4g; Chol 8mg; Sodium 514mg

Teriyaki Steak Fingers

Serves 8

Ingredients

2 pounds sirloin steak, trimmed

½ cup light soy sauce

¼ cup vinegar

2 tablespoons brown sugar

2 tablespoons minced onion

1 tablespoon canola oil

1 tablespoon minced garlic

½ teaspoon ground ginger

¼ teaspoon pepper

8 wooden skewers

Directions

1. Soak skewers in water for 20 minutes. Set aside.

2. Cut steak into ½-inch strips; place in a large bowl.

3. Add the vinegar, brown sugar, onion, oil, garlic, ginger, and pepper to the bowl; mix well. Cover and refrigerate at least 2 hours.

4. Thread meat onto skewers and grill 3 to 5 minutes.

Calories 169 (37% from fat); Fat 7g (sat 2g); Protein 21g; Carb 4g; Fiber 0g; Chol 60mg; Sodium 951mg

Dinner

81

Better-than-Pizza Potatoes

Serves 4

Ingredients

4 medium baking potatoes, baked

¼ teaspoon oregano

¼ cup chopped red and green bell peppers

4 teaspoons dried butter substitute

¼ cup canned diced tomatoes, drained

salt and pepper, to taste

4 tablespoons shredded low-fat Mozzarella cheese

Directions

1 Preheat oven to 350°F.

2 Slice off tops of potato and scoop out flesh, leaving ¼ inch of skin on each side.

3 In a medium bowl, combine the potato flesh, oregano, green and red bell peppers, butter substitute, tomatoes, and salt and pepper.

4 Spoon mixture into the shells and top with cheese. Bake 10 minutes, or until heated through. These can also be heated in a microwave for 2 to 3 minutes.

Calories 198 (8% from fat); Fat 2g (sat 1g); Protein 6g; Carb 40g; Fiber 4g; Chol 6mg; Sodium 74mg

Walk
the
Weight
Away!

Cheesy Broccoli Gratin

Serves 8

Ingredients

4 ½ cups day-old white bread, crusts removed, cut into ½-inch cubes

6 tablespoons dried butter substitute, divided

½ teaspoon chili powder

½ teaspoon garlic powder

1 teaspoon prepared yellow mustard

2 cups nonfat milk

20 ounces frozen broccoli florets, thawed

Directions

1 Preheat oven to 400°F. Spray a 13-by-9-inch baking pan with non-stick cooking spray.

2 In a large bowl, combine the bread cubes, 4 tablespoons of the butter substitute, the chili powder, and the garlic powder.

3 In a small bowl, combine the mustard and the milk. Pour mixture over bread cubes; let sit 5 minutes.

4 Arrange broccoli florets in baking dish. Pour bread mixture onto broccoli and sprinkle with remaining butter substitute.

5 Bake 30 to 40 minutes, until golden brown and bubbly.

Calories 131 (11% from fat); Fat 2g (sat 1g); Protein 6g; Carb 23g; Fiber 2g; Chol 5mg; Sodium 213mg

Grilled Eggplant Wedges

Serves 8

Ingredients

¼ cup olive oil

1 ½ teaspoon garlic powder

1 eggplant, cut into 16 wedges

Directions

1 Preheat countertop grill.

2 In a small bowl, combine the garlic powder and olive oil.

3 Brush mixture onto wedges and grill 2 to 3 minutes, turning once.

Calories 21 (23% from fat); Fat 1g (sat 0g); Protein 1g; Carb 4g; Fiber 1g; Chol 0mg; Sodium 2mg

Grilled Pineapple Slices

Serves 2

Ingredients

1 15-ounce can sliced pineapple, drained

1 tablespoon brown sugar

butter-flavored cooking spray

Directions

1 Preheat grill pan or countertop grill.

2 Coat each pineapple slice with a little cooking spray and top with a little brown sugar.

3 Grill slices for 1 minute.

4 Serve over frozen yogurt or alone.

Calories 86 (3% from fat); Fat 0g (sat 0g); Protein 1g; Carb 22g; Fiber 2g; Chol 0mg; Sodium 4mg

Side
Dishes

85

Nutty Balsamic Green Beans

Serves 4

Ingredients

1 pound fresh green beans, trimmed and washed

⅛ cup chopped walnuts

¼ cup chopped onion

¼ cup broth (any variety)

2 tablespoons balsamic vinegar

Directions

1 In a medium saucepan, steam the beans until bright green; drain and set aside.

2 Heat walnuts in a dry, heavy skillet over medium heat for 1 to 2 minutes or until golden brown and fragrant.

2 Transfer nuts to a bowl, wipe skillet and add 1 teaspoon olive oil. Add onions and sauté until tender, about 3 minutes.

3 Add the broth and vinegar to the onions in the skillet. Add green beans and cook until most of the liquid has evaporated.

4 Transfer beans to a serving bowl, toss with nuts and serve.

Calories 131 (11% from fat); Fat 2g (sat 1g); Protein 6g; Carb 23g; Fiber 2g; Chol 5mg; Sodium 213mg

Walk
the
Weight
Away!

Rice Pilaf

Serves 6

Ingredients

1 tablespoon olive oil

½ cup long-grain rice

½ cup chopped scallion

½ cup chopped red bell pepper

¼ cup dry white wine

3 teaspoons vinegar, divided

1 ¼ teaspoon lemon pepper spice blend, divided

½ cup frozen peas

1 medium zucchini, diced

Directions

1 Heat the oil in a medium skillet set over medium heat.

2 Add the rice, scallion, and red bell pepper. Sauté, stirring constantly, until rice is golden.

3 Gradually stir in the wine, 2 teaspoons of vinegar, 1 teaspoon of lemon pepper spice blend, and 1 cup hot water.

4 Bring mixture to a boil, reduce heat, and add the peas and zucchini.

5 Simmer, covered, until vegetables are tender. Remove from heat.

6 Sprinkle with remaining vinegar and lemon pepper spice blend; fluff with a fork and serve.

Calories 65 (35% from fat); Fat 3g (sat 0g); Protein 2g; Carb 8g; Fiber 2g; Chol 0mg; Sodium 113mg

Chapter 3

The *Walk the Weight Away!* Nutrition Plan

Roasted Carrots with Lime

Serves 8

Ingredients

1 ½ pounds carrots, peeled and cut into thin diagonal slices

2 tablespoons fresh lime juice

6 tablespoons dark or light brown sugar

1 teaspoon garlic powder

1 teaspoon herb blend of your choice

lime wedges, for garnish

Directions

1 Preheat oven to 375°F.

2 Coat a 9- x 13-inch baking pan with non-stick cooking spray.

3 Arrange carrots in a single layer in the dish; sprinkle with lime juice and 2 tablespoons of water.

4 In a small bowl, combine brown sugar, garlic powder, and herbs. Mix well and sprinkle onto the carrots.

5 Bake, covered, for 20 minutes. Uncover pan and turn carrots to coat on all sides. Return to oven and bake, uncovered, until carrots are tender, glazed, and slightly brown, 5 to 10 minutes more.

Calories 68 (2% from fat); Fat 0g (sat 0g); Protein 1g; Carb 17g; Fiber 3g; Chol 0mg; Sodium 63mg

Smashed Potatoes

Serves 4

Ingredients

4 Yukon gold potatoes, cut into 1-inch cubes

1 teaspoon butter

½ cup liquid non-fat, non-dairy creamer

1 tablespoon pepper

1 tablespoon parsley flakes

Directions

1 Cook the potatoes in a large pot of water until tender. Drain and return to pot.

2 Add butter to the potatoes.

3 Warm the creamer in the microwave on MEDIUM for 10 to 15 seconds and add to the pot.

4 Add the pepper and parsley flakes and stir well.

5 Mash the potatoes with a masher; serve.

Calories 210 (26% from fat); Fat 6g (sat 1g); Protein 4g; Carb 35g; Fiber 2g; Chol 3mg; Sodium 361mg

Side
Dishes

89

Chapter 3
The *Walk the Weight Away!* Nutrition Plan

Spinach Salad

Serves 4

Ingredients

1 pound raw spinach, washed well and drained

1 tablespoon olive oil

½ cup bacon bits

½ cup chopped red onion

½ cup vinegar

1 teaspoon sugar

¼ teaspoon dried mustard

¼ teaspoon black pepper

Directions

1 In a large serving bowl, combine the spinach and olive oil and toss well.

2 In a small bowl, combine the bacon bits, onion, vinegar, sugar, mustard, and pepper. Mix well.

3 Pour dressing over spinach, toss, and serve.

Calories 77 (33% from fat); Fat 3g (sat 0g); Protein 4g; Carb 11g; Fiber 3g; Chol 0mg; Sodium 98mg

Thai Pasta Salad

Serves 4

Ingredients

6 ounces silken tofu

¼ cup peanut butter

2 tablespoons vinegar

2 tablespoons light soy sauce

2 tablespoons sugar

2 teaspoons ginger

1 teaspoon sesame oil

¼ teaspoon cayenne pepper

1 clove garlic, minced

1 cup fresh green soybeans

½ pound snow peas, cut in 1-inch pieces

1 red bell pepper, chopped

1 cup broccoli florets

2 carrots, thinly sliced

8 ounces vermicelli, broken in half

¼ cup chopped scallions

Directions

1 For the dressing, place the tofu, peanut butter, vinegar, soy sauce, sugar, ginger, oil, cayenne, garlic, and ¾ cup water in the pitcher of a blender. Process until smooth; refrigerate.

2 For the salad, place the soybeans in a medium saucepan. Cover with water; simmer until tender, about 15 minutes. Fill another large saucepan with water; bring to a boil. Blanch the snow peas, red bell pepper, broccoli, and carrots for 1 minute. Drain.

3 Cook vermicelli according to package directions. Drain, rinse and toss with soybeans and vegetables. Refrigerate at least 2 hours.

4 Just before serving, toss with dressing and top with scallions.

Calories 502 (27% from fat); Fat 15g (sat 3g); Protein 26g; Carb 71g; Fiber 9g; Chol 0mg; Sodium 593mg

Side Dishes

Chapter 3

The *Walk the Weight Away!* Nutrition Plan

Waldorf Salad

Serves 2

Ingredients

1 tablespoon lemon juice

1 tablespoon orange juice

1 teaspoon sugar

2 tablespoons non-fat milk

⅓ cup low-fat mayonnaise

2 apples (any variety), cored and cut into cubes

3 celery stalks, chopped

½ cup raisins

½ cup walnuts

Directions

1 In large bowl combine the juices, sugar, milk, and mayonnaise; mix well.

2 Add the apple cubes, celery, raisins, and walnuts. Toss and serve.

Calories 367 (28% from fat); Fat 11g (sat 1g); Protein 6g; Carb 69g; Fiber 9g; Chol 5mg; Sodium 386mg

Walk
the
Weight
Away!

Putting It All Together

Now that we've reviewed some of the basic information on nutrition and covered topics including healthful recipes and how eating well can help you lose weight, you're ready to learn more about your walking workout program.

While it's true that you could lose weight through dieting alone, research has shown over and over that it is the combination of exercise and weight loss that leads to permanent (and faster) results. So get ready to put on your walking shoes and hit the pavement, the track, or the treadmill. This is an exciting lifestyle change you are about to embark on, and one that may come with some challenges. It is always difficult to break a habit, whether it be a sedentary lifestyle or fondness for junk food. Before we set out on our walk, let's take a look at what happens when you make major changes to your lifestyle and what you need to know to optimize your success.

93

Starting a Brand New Journey

You are beginning a new journey on the road to a healthier, happier weight and a fit lifestyle. In the past you may have been the type of person who didn't pay attention to what you ate. Lots of busy people are like this. They eat on the run (literally—in their cars, and on trains). Such habits may cause you to eat foods that are high in calories and low in nutritional value. You may also spend most of your leisure time (the little of it that there is) watching TV. Or, you may be used to driving everywhere—even to a store that is only a few blocks from your home. In other words, the new eating and walking plans that you are about to embrace in *Walk the Weight Away!* may be markedly different from what you have been used to. And this will pose somewhat of a challenge as you change your behavior.

Using Our Nutrition Guide

To make sure that you get the most out of this program, it is important to understand the "whys" of your behaviors as well as the "whats." What do we mean by this? Well, the "whats" might be the kinds of foods you eat; the "whys"—why you ate them at a given time. Were you depressed? Happy? Sad? Frustrated? If you keep track of your eating and exercising habits, you can determine your emotional and physical triggers both for healthful and not-so-healthful eating patterns. Take another look at the sample Nutrition Guide on page 44, which is reproduced in Part II of this book for an eight-week time period. In this diary you can record what, when, and where you eat, and how you're feeling as you eat. Keeping a food diary will help you track your eating patterns and identify behaviors you may want to change.

In your diary you may also want to note what you were doing when you ate (were you watching TV, talking on the phone?). This information will provide you with clues about your eating habits, and help you avoid high-risk situations in the future. You will also record your walking progress, which can also be found in the workbook section of this book.

Psychology of Starting Something New

Experts recognize that the best way to successfully change your diet and exercise behavior is to take an approach that includes nutritional counseling, an exercise program, and a psychological component. What does psychology have to do with something so distinctly physical? Well, like most things in life our minds and bodies are intricately connected. Weight loss research has shown that in order to change your body, you must first adjust your mind-set. Remember, your goal is a new lifestyle—not a quick-fix diet plan. Here are some things you should know about the psychology of starting something new.

It's About Attitude

The first thing you need to do is adjust your attitudes and beliefs. Look inward to fully understand why you may overeat or why you don't exercise. Perhaps you are an emotional eater who eats when you are angry, depressed, or even happy. Or, you may be a lazy eater who just reaches for the closest and easiest food. You may not exercise because you feel that you are no good at it, that it will be too difficult, or because you simply hate it.

Answer the following questions:

1. How many times have you tried to lose weight or exercise?
2. How long have results lasted?
3. Why did you gain back the weight or stop exercising?
4. How did you feel when you gained back the weight?
5. Are you confident that you can achieve your weight-loss goals?
6. Do you believe that you can commit to changing your lifestyle so that your results will last your whole life?

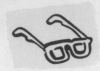

Don't let past failures stand in the way of a healthy future—no matter what your past experiences with diet and exercise have been, you are capable of tremendous change.

Walk the Weight Away!

The answers to these questions provide you with a baseline assessment of your current attitudes and beliefs about weight loss. They make clear how you feel, right now, about your prior weight loss attempts. If you answered that you felt like a failure when you gained back the weight, you need to acknowledge that feeling (because as a feeling it is valid and needs to be recognized) but then you need to set it aside. People are capable of tremendous, amazing changes in their lives, regardless of their pasts.

Having the confidence and ability to avoid temptation when faced with difficult situations is called self-efficacy by social researchers. People need to have high levels of self-efficacy—they need to believe in their capacity for success—in order to succeed. It's like in the children's story The Little Engine that Could. Just like the little engine in that story, you need to believe in your abilities, even when the going gets rough.

Change Occurs in Stages

Research has established that behavioral change is not a cut and dry event—it is a process that unfolds over time. One of the most respected and widely followed theories of behavioral change is The Stages of Change, developed by the researchers Prochaska and DiClemente. They proposed that all changes in behavior involve cycling through a series of stages of readiness to change. Initially, this model was applied to smokers who were trying to kick the habit. Prochaska and DiClemente found that smokers changed their behavior (stopped smoking) through a series of stages. At each stage, there were certain mental and behavioral strategies that helped them move on to the next stage.

This stage model of change has been adapted to cover a wide range of health behaviors including diet and exercise. The model states that change involves progressing through the following five stages: precontemplation, contemplation, preparation, action, and maintenance. It is not uncommon for people to go through the cycle a few times before they can make their change permanent. That's just part of the process. Take the time to determine which stage you are in with regard to weight loss or exercise.

Precontemplation. You do not plan to change your behavior; in fact, you are very unmotivated and resistant to change. It is highly unlikely, as a reader of this book, that you are in this first stage. Congratulations! You are at the very least in the next stage, Contemplation.

Contemplation. You are seriously thinking about changing your behavior. In fact you intend to change within six months. You want to lose the weight and start exercising because you believe it is important for your health and quality of life. But, you may be plagued by negative thoughts at this stage. You are worried about how much time you'll need to spend exercising, or whether you will be able to follow a healthy eating plan.

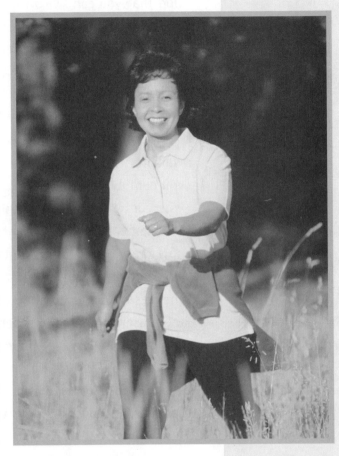

If you are at this stage, we will help you address your concerns so that you can move on to the next stage. Now is also the time to consider some unexpected sources of resistance to change.

Do you feel helpless and hopeless about your prospects? Maybe this is an attitude that blocks you in many aspects of your life. Learn to activate the virtue of hope.

Do you secretly like being overweight? Maybe you identify with celebrities who are heavy. Perhaps it makes you feel important, like you stand out in a crowd.

Are you afraid to be thin? Maybe your heaviness has protected you against being hurt by others. Learn to handle emotional issues psychologically, the way they should be handled, instead of physically.

Do you think you will lose friends by getting in shape? Chances are you will become a model for many of your friends who are also struggling with too much body fat.

Are you afraid of being too attractive if you are slim, maybe even too sexually attractive? If you are, give thought to what conflicts exist here and try to resolve them in a healthier way.

Will being thin mean that you will have to throw out your favorite clothes and buy new ones? Well, that's part of the price you'll have to pay for being a healthier, happier person.

Chapter 4
Starting a Brand New Journey

When you're trying to change your behavior it's important to remember that an occasional slip-up is to be expected. Consider it just a temporary setback and get right back on track again the next day.

Do you fear that the 'real you' will disappear? Are you worried that the fun-loving overweight person who loved to carouse and was the butt of jokes will become so thin that he or she won't be visible any more? You will find that you can live with that and that the light of your true personality will shine through no matter what your size.

Preparation. You are ready to take action in the immediate future. You are highly motivated and have a positive attitude about your ability to change. You are ready to go. If you are at this stage, you are ready to set your goals and begin to *Walk the Weight Away!*

Action. You are immersed in your behavior change. Once you begin your walking program, you will be in action. During this stage we recommend that you continue to use self-monitoring and stimulus control in order to ensure your continued success in the maintenance stage.

Maintenance. Maintenance means you have reached your goals and now are working to prevent a relapse or temporary slip. You can prevent relapse by avoiding high-risk situations (those situations that increase the chances of your overeating or not exercising—for example wandering down the dessert aisle at the supermarket). If you should suffer a slip, think of it as what it is—just a temporary setback—and get right back on track again the next day. Ask yourself what you have learned from the experience, and use that knowledge to avoid future slips. Remain calm, and then renew your commitment to your new eating and exercise plan.

Walk
the
Weight
Away!

Exercise Basics

As you work through the program in this book you will be engaging in aerobic conditioning, one of the three pillars of fitness training. The other two are strength training and flexibility training. You may be wondering if you really need to bother with strength and flexibility training. After all, you just want to shed some pounds, and we've already established that walking is an effective calorie burner. So why bother with the other two? The answer is simple. Yes, you can lose weight with just a walking program, but if you want to lose weight more efficiently, be more fit, and prevent injury, you need to also incorporate strength and flexibility training. You can think of each fitness pillar as an angle on a triangle. The triangle represents a person who is fully fit, one who has muscular strength, flexibility, and aerobic conditioning. Each pillar influences the other. For example, the more flexible you are the better your walking stride will be; and the stronger your legs are, the more power and endurance you will have for your walk. Let's take a look at each pillar in detail.

Aerobic Conditioning

Our bodies produce energy in our cells; this energy is known as adenosine triphosphate, or ATP and it is the fuel that provides energy for activity. ATP can be produced in a variety of ways, one of which is through the aerobic system. Strictly speaking, the aerobic energy system uses oxygen, fatty acids, and glucose to produce energy. When you exercise intensely over a long enough period of time, you are helping your body burn fat, which creates energy and burns calories.

Aerobic conditioning involves rhythmically moving large muscle groups, at the right intensity, continuously for at least 20 to 30 minutes. Moving large muscles is necessary to increase blood flow (and therefore oxygen) throughout the body and back to the heart. It is this increase in blood flow that strengthens the heart, making it a more effective and healthier pumping muscle. Examples of aerobic conditioning activities include walking, running, swimming, aerobics, and biking. All are good ways to increase your cardiovascular fitness.

We mentioned that when you do aerobic exercise, your body burns fat in order to create energy. Therefore, this type of exercise will help you lose weight. In general, your body goes into fat-burning mode after about 20 minutes of aerobic exercise, which is why this is the recommended minimum duration for an aerobic exercise session. The American College of Sports Medicine has issued the following guidelines for healthy aerobic activity:

- Exercise three to five days each week (at least five if weight-loss is your goal)
- Warm up for 5 to 10 minutes before starting the aerobic activity.
- Maintain your exercise intensity for 30 to 45 minutes and then gradually decrease the intensity of your work out before cooling down.

As you exercise, your heart rate increases to meet your body's increased demand for blood and oxygen. The greater the intensity of your workout, the faster your heart will beat. Exercising at the right intensity is crucial for your aerobic workout. If you work out at too low an intensity, you will not be burning fat, and if you work out at too high an intensity, you may over strain your system. The safest and most effective intensities for working out are represented in a range of heart rates, known as your training zone.

Gauging The Intensity of Your Aerobic Exercise

There are several different ways to estimate your training zone, but the most common, and simplest is the following formula. First, estimate your maximal heart rate (the fastest your heart can beat) by subtracting your age from 220. So, if you're 40 years old:

220 − 40 = 180

Multiply the result first by 50 percent to find the lower end of your target heart rate range and then by 80 percent to find the upper end. Again, if you're 40 years old:

180 x .5 = 90 beats per minute
180 x .8 = 144 beats per minute.

In this example, the exerciser should keep her heart rate between 90 and 144 to reap the benefits of aerobic exercise.

If math isn't your favorite subject, don't worry, because the chart on page 102 will tell you exactly what your heart rate range ought to be.

If you're new to aerobic exercise, and have been pretty sedentary, you should work out at the lower end of your zone and gradually build up. The more fit your cardiorespiratory system becomes, the more intense you can make your workouts. Years ago, people thought that it was better to work out for very long periods of time at the low end of their zone, believing that this was the most effective way to burn fat. In fact, research has shown that for best results (both in terms of weight loss and benefits to your cardiovascular health) it is preferable to work out at the higher intensities—so long as they are appropriate for you, given your conditioning level and any health issues. Be sensible about interpreting all this information though. If you haven't gotten off the couch for years and are extremely out of shape, then you want to go easy at first, stay in the low end, and maybe accumulate your 20 or 30 minutes throughout the day rather than in one continuous shot.

The best way to gauge your workout intensity is with a heart rate monitor, which gives a pretty accurate reading in beats per minute. Alternatively, you can take your heart rate at a number of pulse sites on your body. One popular site is the wrist. Place your index and middle finger over the under-

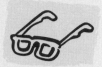

If you've been sedentary for years and are extremely out of shape, start off slow and go easy. Stay in the lower end of your target heart range and accumulate your 20 or 30 minutes throughout the day rather than in one intense workout.

101

Heart Rate Ranges for Aerobic Exercise

Age	220-age	50%	80%	Age	220-age	50%	80%
80	140	70	112	52	168	84	134
79	141	71	113	51	169	85	135
78	142	71	114	50	170	85	136
77	143	72	114	49	171	86	137
76	144	72	115	48	172	86	138
75	145	73	116	47	173	87	138
74	146	73	117	46	174	87	139
73	147	74	118	45	175	88	140
72	148	74	118	44	176	88	141
71	149	75	119	43	177	89	142
70	150	75	120	42	178	89	142
69	151	76	121	41	179	90	143
68	152	76	122	40	180	90	144
67	153	77	122	39	181	91	145
66	154	77	123	38	182	91	146
65	155	78	124	37	183	92	146
64	156	78	125	36	184	92	147
63	157	79	126	35	185	93	148
62	158	79	126	34	186	93	149
61	159	80	127	33	187	94	150
60	160	80	128	32	188	94	150
59	161	81	129	31	189	95	151
58	162	81	130	30	190	95	152
57	163	82	130	29	191	96	153
56	164	82	131	28	192	96	154
55	165	83	132	27	193	97	154
54	166	83	133	26	194	97	155
53	167	84	134	25	195	98	156

Walk
the
Weight
Away!

side of the opposite wrist, below the base of the thumb. Press firmly until you feel the pulse. Once you find the pulse, count the beats for 1 full minute, or for 30 seconds and multiply by 2. This will give the beats per minute. Use two fingers of one hand to locate the carotid artery (in your neck) and begin counting your pulse, starting with zero for 10 seconds. Multiply that number by 6. This method is much less reliable than using a heart rate monitor, and the results can vary depending on the amount of pressure you're placing on your neck and the accuracy of your counting.

Another way to gauge intensity (and one that can be used as a complement to calculating heart rate) is with the rating of perceived exertion (also called the Borg Scale). This scale uses how you feel while exercising as a way to determine if you are working too hard or not hard enough. Because it requires no calculation and no equipment, it is extremely easy to do. The scale ranges from 6 to 20 and represents the amount of effort you feel you are expending (see chart). Doing nothing (sitting down) would be a 6, "noth-

ing at all"; walking at a very brisk pace might be a 3, "moderate" or 4, "somewhat strong." For aerobic conditioning you want your perceived exertion rating to stay between 12 and 14.

Whenever you are doing aerobic conditioning, you should feel able to carry on a conversation during your

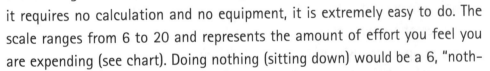

RATING PERCEIVED EXERTION

6	No exertion at all
7	Extremely light (7.5)
8, 9	Very light
10,11	Light
12,13	Somewhat hard
14, 15	Hard (heavy)
16, 17	Very hard
18, 19	Extremely hard
20	Maximal exertion

workout (this is called the Talk Test), even if it takes a bit of effort. Never work out to the point of feeling dizzy, faint, or like you might collapse from exhaustion.

Flexibility Training

How often do you hear someone (or maybe even yourself) complain about tightness in the lower back or legs? What can be done about it? All too often, in our rush to burn calories and fat, we neglect flexibility training, despite the fact that it is an important component of fitness and it is well worth the extra few minutes a day that it takes. A regular stretching routine helps improve your range of motion; it makes your body feel less tight and more nimble. If you don't stretch your muscles, you are more likely to get injured and your workouts, including your walks, will suffer. Stretched muscles also develop that nice long, lean look that dancers have. And, as a bonus, because it emphasizes deep breathing, stretching is a great way to relax and relieve tension (try stretching to some soothing music in a dimly lit room or out in a garden).

Stretching is essential both before and after your walk. Before your walk, you will engage in what is known as active stretching or an active warm-up, which basically means you perform a less intense version of your walk. So, if you are going to walk at a 15 minute per mile pace, your warm up would be about 5 minutes at a slower pace, for example, 20 minutes per mile. The purpose of the warm up stretch is to prepare your body for your workout—to get the blood flowing through your legs and arms, and to slightly elevate your heart rate. People used to do static stretches (stretches where you just hold a stretch position for a number of seconds) before walking or running, but research has shown no benefit to static stretching before a workout. In fact, if your muscles are cold, too much of a stretch may actually tear the muscle.

After your walk is when you will do your static stretches (a program of static stretches is presented at the end of this chapter.) Why? Because at the end of your workout, your muscles are warm—your heart has been pumping blood to those working muscles to deliver oxygen to them. Muscles are more flexile when they are warm—they can be stretched more safely, and effectively. Optimally, a static stretch should be held for 20 seconds (the minimum amount of time is 10 seconds).

Strength Training

The benefits of strength training have been getting loads of press these days. For good reason; it works wonders. Talk to anyone who has incorporated weight training—using additional resistance to challenge or overload your muscles—into their fitness program and they will tell you how their bodies truly changed after they began to use weights. The reasons are plentiful. *Number one:* thanks to gravity's downward pull, your body starts to lose muscle at the rate of approximately 1/2 pound a year beginning at around age 30. Muscle tone is what gives our bodies their shapes—the contours are all due to how firm we are, not how thin we are. If you keep losing muscle over the years, you will lose shape, and will have hanging skin. *Number two:* When muscles are overloaded, they get stronger and your percentage of lean body mass increases, while your percentage of body fat decreases. *Number three:* Muscle burns more calories at rest than fat; if you have more lean body mass, you *will burn more calories when doing absolutely nothing* (your resting metabolism will rise) than someone who weighs as much as you, but has less muscle. *Number four:* You will have more strength to do things in everyday life, such as pushing heavy doors or carrying bags of groceries. *Number five:* Your risk of injury will decrease because you are stronger. *And lastly:* Strength training can help prevent or treat osteoporosis, the prevalent thinning bone disease, by increasing bone density.

With all these great reasons to do strength training, how could you not? Especially when research has shown that everyone at any age (even people well into their nineties) can benefit from a strength-training program. The beautiful thing about strength training is that you only have to do it a couple of times a week for about 15 to 20 minutes each time to get results. Ask yourself if you have an extra 30 or 40 minutes a week to be stronger, sleeker, leaner, and healthier. You will find a sample strengthening program, which describes how to strength train effectively, at the end of the chapter.

Stretch and Strengthen

As we've said, the three main pillars of fitness are cardiovascular fitness, flexibility, and muscular strength and endurance. For optimal fitness, you should do activities that target each of these areas. Therefore, the following stretching and strengthening routines are provided to complement your walking program. Stretching and strength training will improve your walking routine by making you stronger and more flexible.

You should do static stretching after every walk and do strength-training exercises at least twice a week beginning in weeks 2 through 4 of your program. Make sure that your form for each exercise is perfect. If possible, perform your exercises in front of a mirror; this will help you see where your form could use improvement.

The Stretching Program

Hold each stretch for a minimum of 10 seconds. Inhale as you begin the stretch; exhale as you execute it. This is a static stretching program, which means you should just hold the stretch as you breathe deeply. Do not bounce. Keep your head in line with your spine. Stretch only to the point of tension, never to pain. As you hold a stretch for a few seconds, the tension should begin to dissipate.

The *Walk the Weight Away!* Stretches

Walk
the
Weight
Away!

Head & Neck Stretch

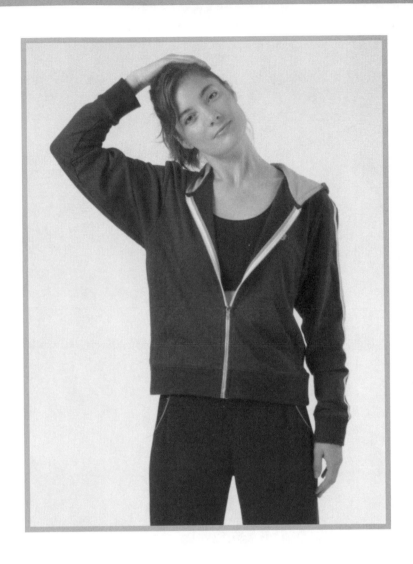

Place your right hand on top of your head and gently press your head toward your right shoulder. Repeat on the other side.

Chapter 5
Exercise Basics

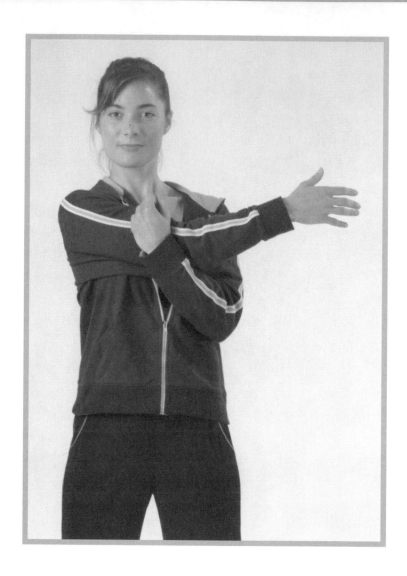

Use your left arm to press your right arm across your body and into your chest. Repeat on the other side.

Walk the **Weight** Away!

Triceps Stretch

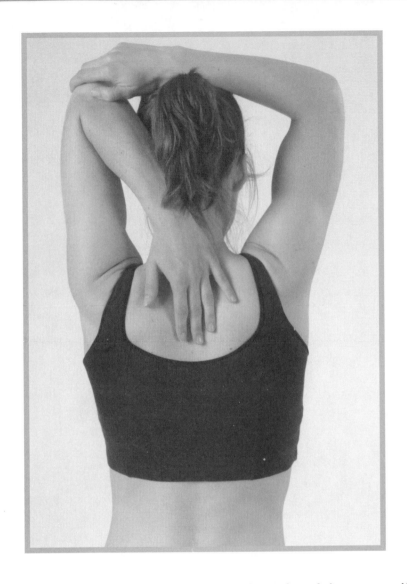

Bend your left arm behind your head, with your elbow facing the ceiling. Use your right arm to press against the left elbow until you feel a stretch in the back of your arm. Repeat on the other side.

Chest & Biceps Stretch

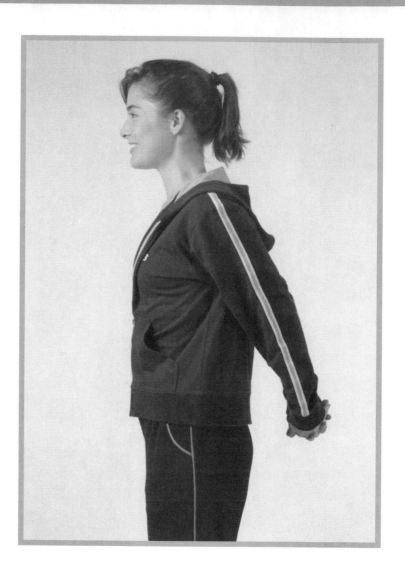

Interlace your fingers behind your back and pull away from your body.

Walk the **Weight** Away!

Upper Back Stretch

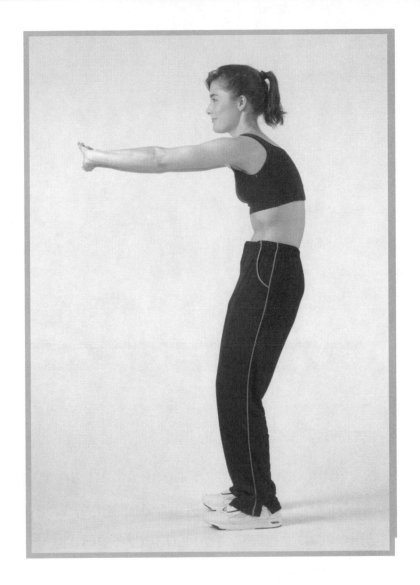

Interlace your fingers, and press your arms out in front of your body, with palms facing outward. Pull your stomach in tight so that your back curves like the letter **C**.

The Egg

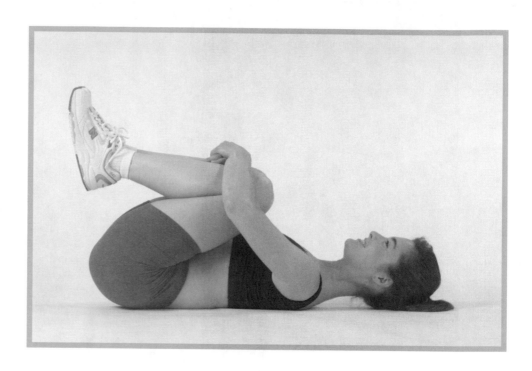

Lay flat on your back on the floor or an an exercise mat. Pull both knees toward your stomach, wrap your arms around your knees, and squeeze gently. Repeat two or three times.

Walk
the
Weight
Away!

Quadriceps Stretch

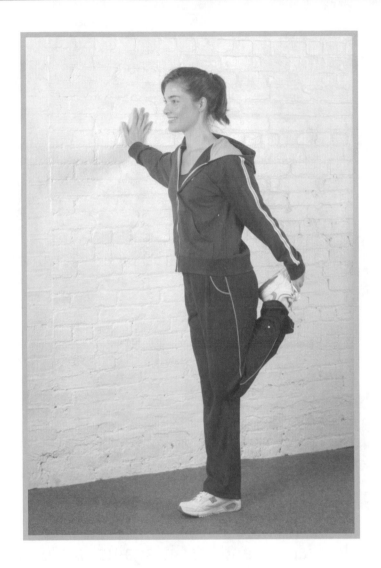

Press your right hand against a wall or other stable surface for balance (if you don't need the support, don't use it). Bend your left leg behind you, holding onto your left ankle with your left hand. Press your heel up and in toward your buttocks. Repeat on the other leg.

Hamstring Stretch

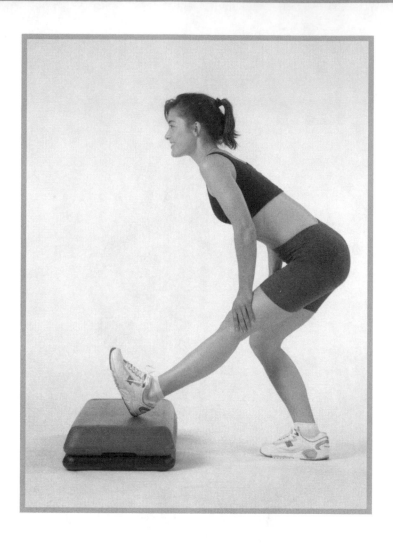

Lift your left leg up and rest it against a step or other surface (how high you go will depend on the flexibility in your hamstrings and lower back). Keep your left leg as straight as you can, bend your right knee, lean forward from the base of your spine, and try to press your chest towards your knee. Repeat on the other leg.

Walk
the
Weight
Away!

Calf Stretch

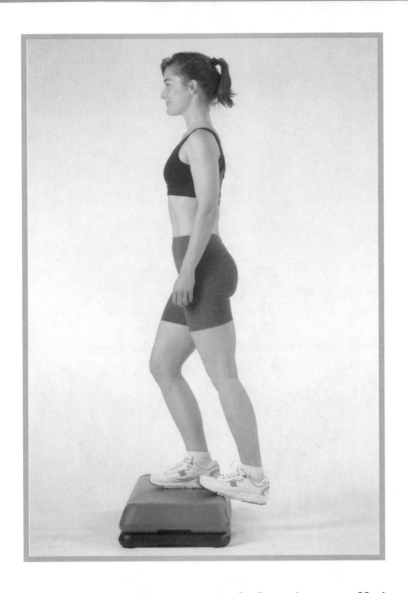

Stand on a step and let your left foot hang off the end. Press down gently but firmly to enhance the stretch in your left calf. Repeat on the other leg.

Butterfly Stretch

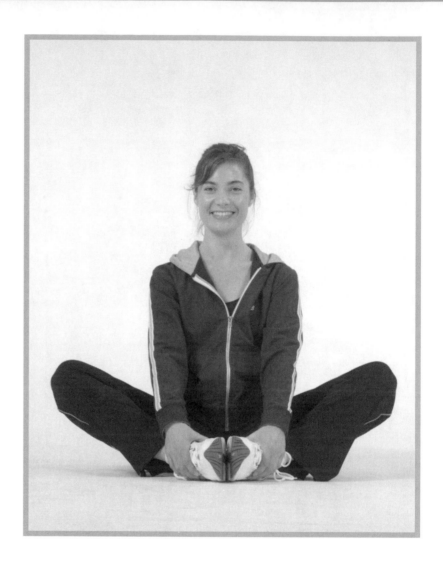

Sit on the floor with your legs bent and the soles of your feet together. Hodling your ankles, slowly and gently push your knees toward the floor, until you feel slight pressure on your inner thigh.

The Strength-Training Program

You will need only hand weights for this strengthening program. Here are the basic guidelines.

- Perform these exercises at least twice a week.
- You don't have to do all of them; aim for at least seven exercises that target different muscle groups, including abdominals. Begin with a single set of 10 to 15 repetitions of each exercise; progress to three sets.
- To build strength you should work to what is called failure (weight training is one the few areas in life where failure equals success). Failure is when you feel like you cannot do another repetition of an exercise without losing your good form (if you are doing a set of 10 reps, you should feel like you are about to hit failure by the eighth rep). If you feel like you can do 20 repetitions easily, this is a signal that you really should be using heavier weights.
- Research has shown that when increasing strength, it is better to perform fewer repetitions with heavier weights than many repetitions with light weights. After a few weeks, increase the weight you are using for resistance by about 10 percent. Remember, you want to continue to challenge and overload your body for best results. For each exercise: lift for two seconds, lower the weight for four seconds.

The *Walk the Weight Away!* **Strength-Training Exercises:**

Chapter 5
Exercise Basics

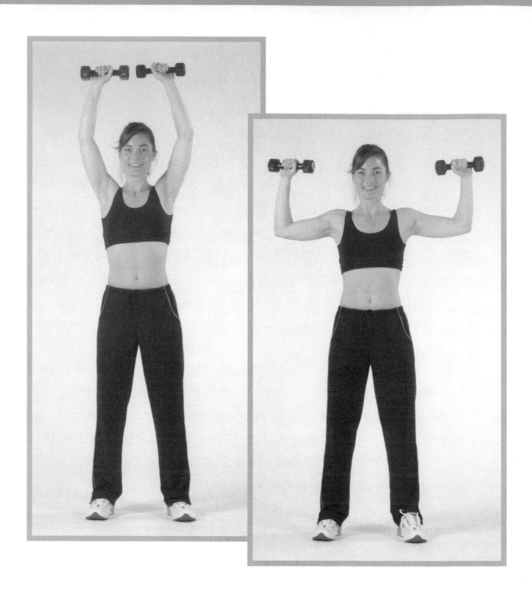

Lift your arms straight overhead (Do not let the weights touch); then bend them back down to the 90-degree start-position.

Walk the **Weight** Away!

Arm Power I

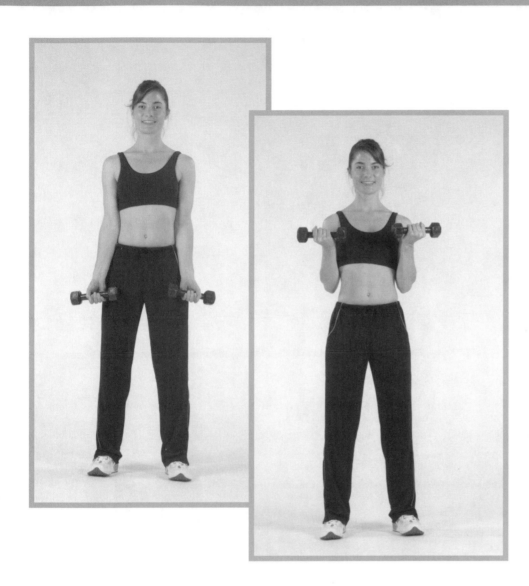

With your palms facing up, and your arms pressed against your sides, curl your arms bringing the weights up to your shoulders. Lower down until you feel a stretch in the front of your arms.

Arm Power II

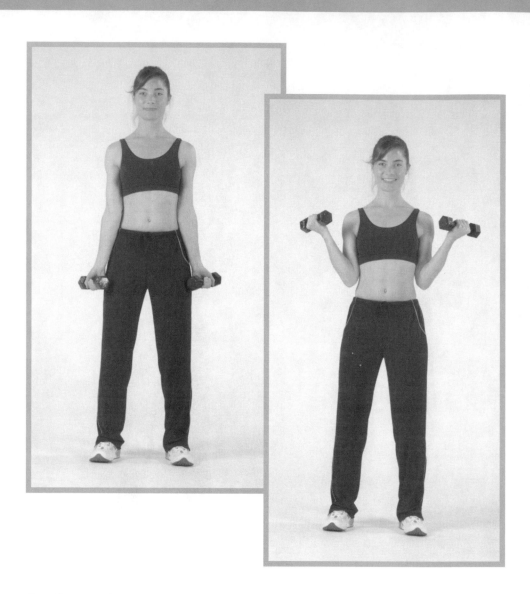

Perform the same exercise, but this time turn your arms out at 45-degree angles and lift and lower.

Walk the **Weight** Away!

Tri Blaster

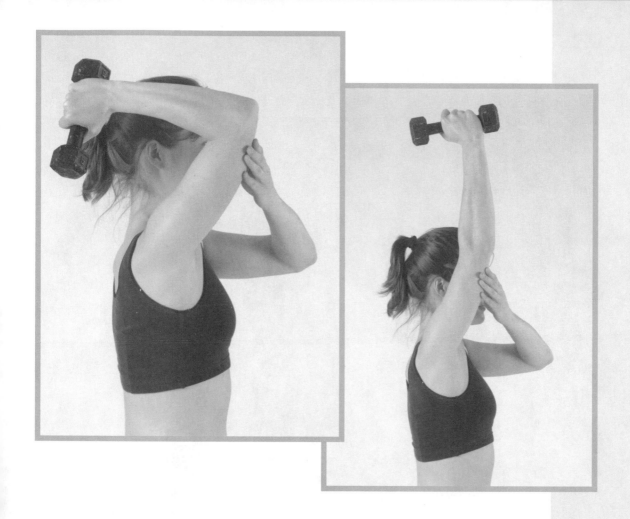

Lift the weight over your head with your elbow pointed at the ceiling. Straighten your arm, slowly bend your elbow, and lower the dumbbell toward your neck. Repeat with the other arm.

121

Back Fly

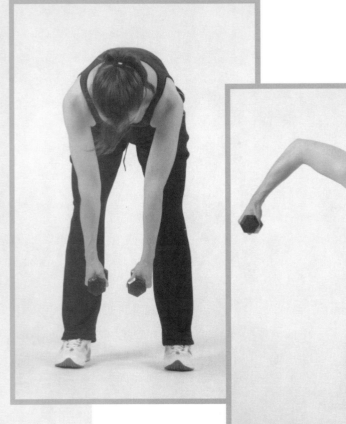

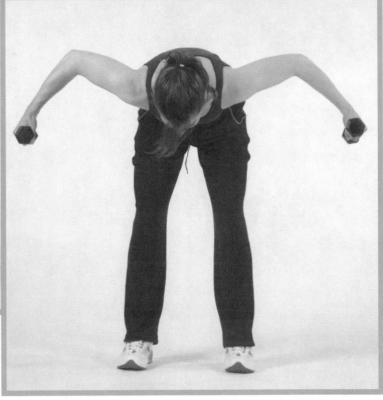

Lean forward from your waist, keeping your head in line with your spine and your knees slightly bent. Begin with the weights together in front of your chest, open up, bringing the weights and your arms out to the side.

Walk
the
Weight
Away!

Modified Push-Up

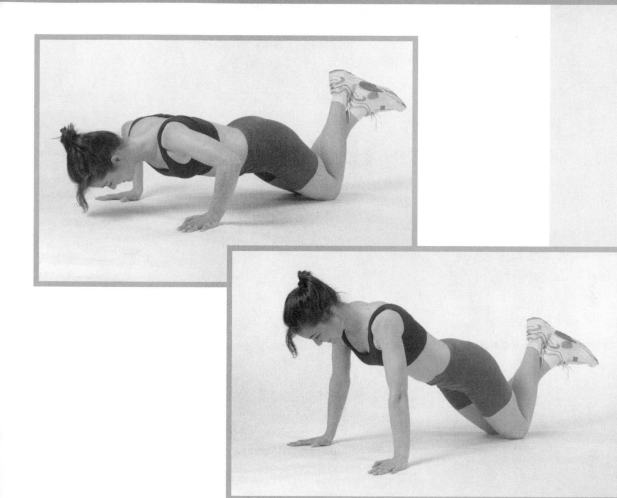

Lie face down on the floor with your knees bent and ankles crossed. With your hands wider than your shoulders perform a push-up, keeping your knees in contact with the floor. Engage your abs as you lift and be sure your back does not sag.

Push-Up

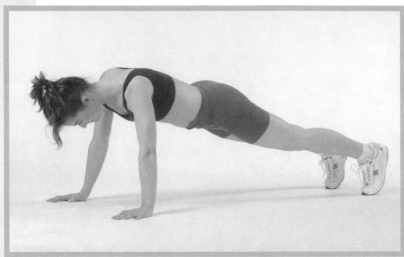

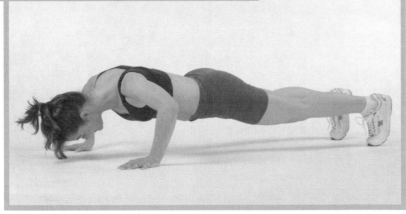

Lie face down on the floor. With your hands wider than your shoulders, perform a push-up, making sure to engage your abs as you lift. Make sure your back does not sag as you lift.

Walk the **Weight** Away!

Front Fly

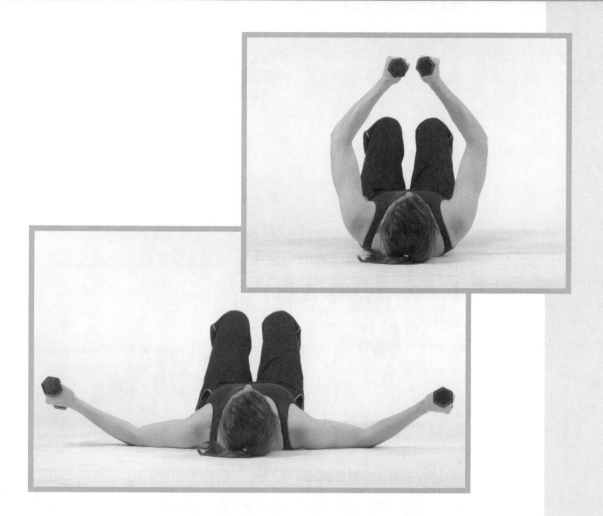

Lie on your back, with your arms out to your sides in an arc. Bring your arms together over your chest, then return back out to your sides until you feel a stretch across your chest.

125

Thigh-Shaper Lunge

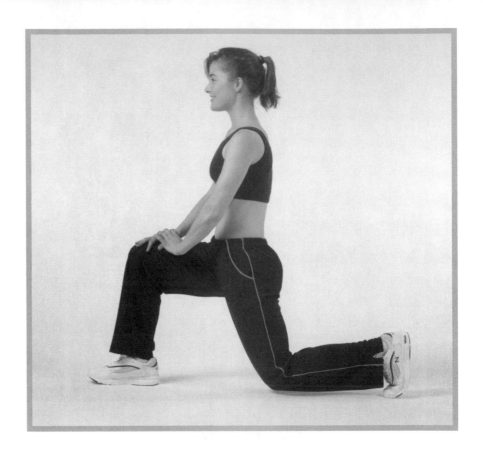

Step forward with your right leg, bending it in front of you to a 90 degree angle. Be careful not to flex your knee forward beyond your ankle. Your back leg should also bend to about a 90 degree angle, with the knee hovering a few inches above the ground. Do several repetitions on one leg, then repeat exercise on the other leg.

Walk
the
Weight
Away!

Best Butt

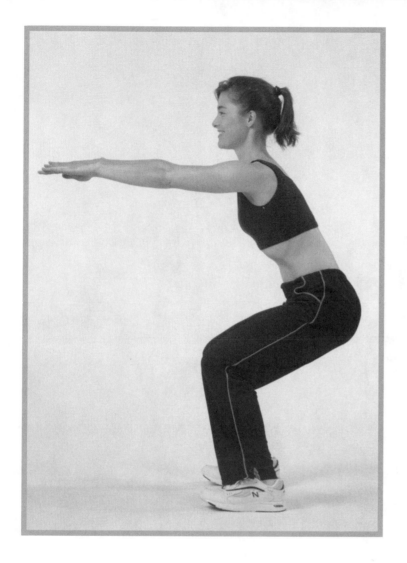

Stand with your legs 12 to 14 inches apart and your knees aligned with your toes. Sit back, as if you are going to sit in a chair that is a foot behind you. Go down as far as parallel to the floor. Pull your stomach muscles in and exhale as you straighten up to the starting position.

Karate Kick

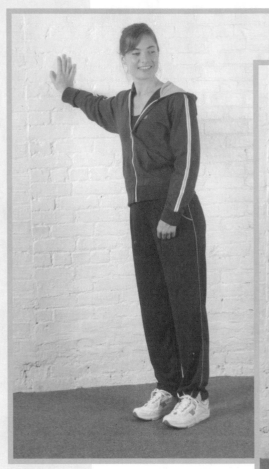

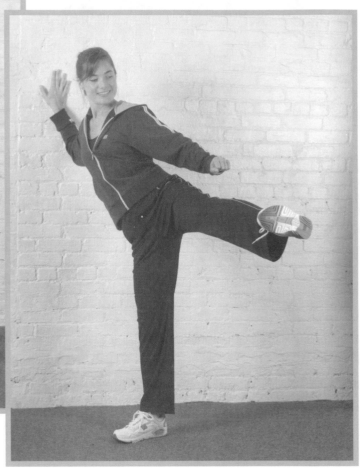

Press your right hand against a wall for support. Kick your left leg out to the side, raising it high enough to feel tension in your outer thigh. Then lower to the starting position. Repeat on the other side.

Walk the **Weight** Away!

Plié Press

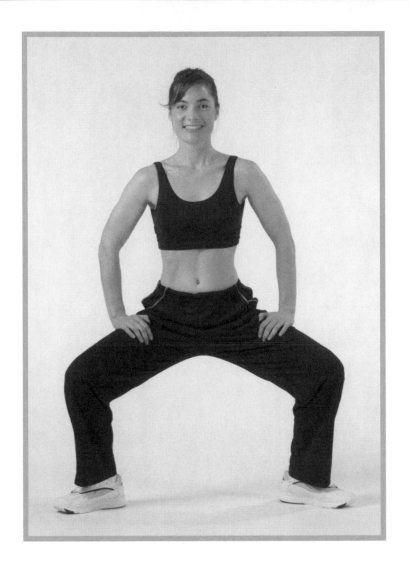

Stand with your legs wide apart, toes pointed to the side. Bend your legs, keeping your knees over your ankles, and then straighten back up to the starting position. Be sure to keep your back perfectly straight as you perform this exercise.

Hot Calves

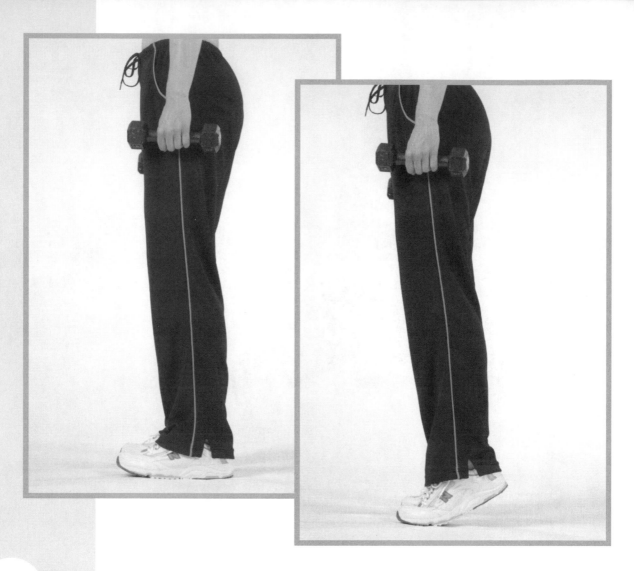

Hold your weights down by your sides; lift onto the balls of your feet and then lower slowly down. You can vary this exercise by turning your toes out or inward to accentuate different parts of your calf.

Walk
the
Weight
Away!

Strong Center

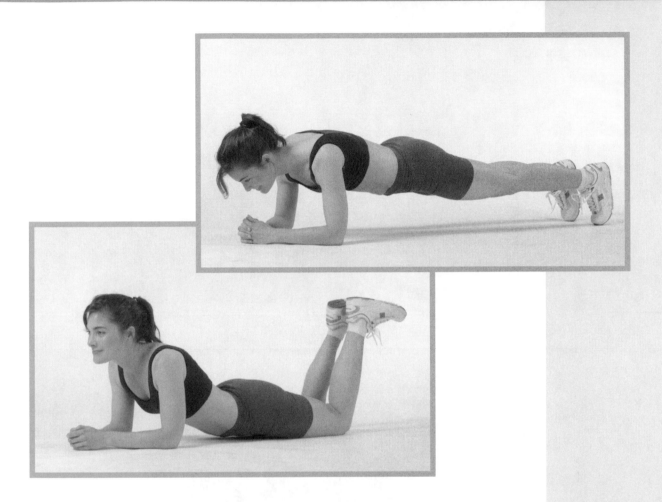

This exercise, known as the plank, will help strengthen your entire core area, including your abdominals, pelvis, and lower back. Place your forearms on the floor and lift your body up, balancing on your forearms and toes. Try to keep your back flat (if you cannot keep it flat in this position, then do the exercise on your hands and knees.) Hold this position for 20 to 30 seconds.

Six Pack

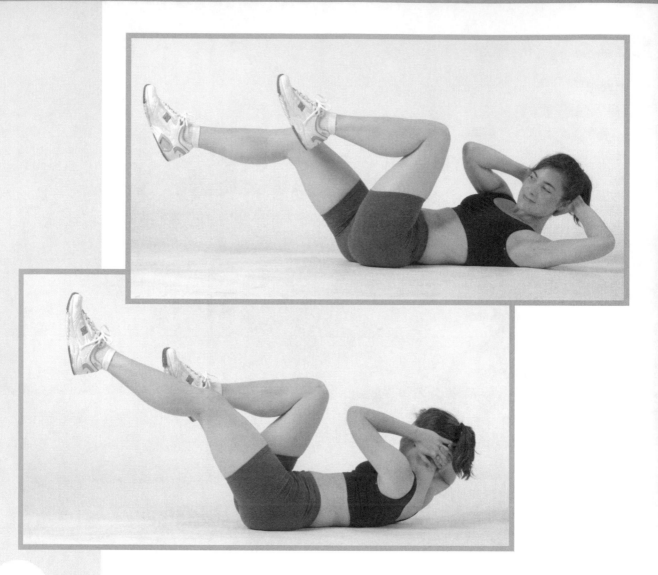

Lie on your back, with your legs up and bent at 90-degree angles. Lift your torso and twist over to one knee as you extend the other leg out; switch to the other side. Perform 16 to 24 repetitions.

Walk
the
Weight
Away!

Basic Crunch

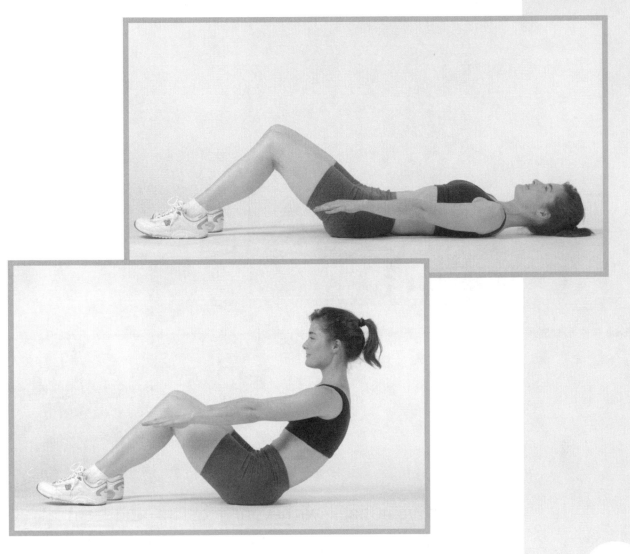

Lie on your back, with your hands either down by your sides or behind your head. Lift your torso, keeping your head in line with your spine, then lower back down without touching your shoulders to the floor. Perform 16 to 24 repetitions.

Crunch Combo

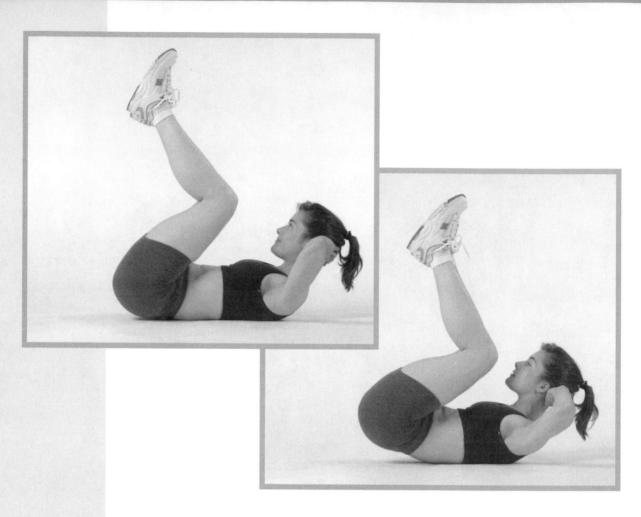

Lie on your back with your legs up and bent at 90 degree angles and your hands behind your head. Lift your tailbone slightly off the floor as you curl your knees toward your torso. At the same time lift your torso to meet your knees. Do this exercise slowly, making sure you don't use your hips to lift your tailbone. Perform 16 to 24 repetitions.

Gearing Up

Now it's time to get ready to walk. Unlike many other types of exercise, walking does not require you to purchase expensive equipment. However, there are certain basics that you will need.

It Starts with the Shoes

First and most important is the proper walking shoe. Anyone who has walked for a half hour on concrete in heels can attest to the fact that while

you can (and do) walk in any shoe, if you are going to walk as a form of exercise you need a shoe that will provide proper cushioning and support to prevent foot injury. Shoes specifically designed for walking are recommended (you can find them in most shoe stores) but you can also use hiking shoes, running shoes, or cross trainers. The right shoe for you depends on the structure of your feet. If you have a high arch, you will need a shoe with greater shock absorption and more lateral support. If you have low arches, you may require less cushioning, greater general support, and heel control.

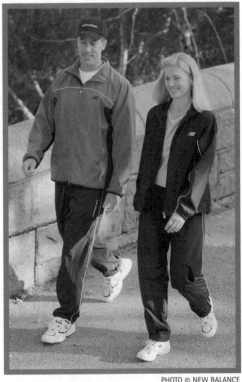

PHOTO © NEW BALANCE

135

FINDING THE PERFECT FIT

- Before you shop for a new pair of shoes, you should have your feet measured for width as well as for length.

- Learn to recognize your foot type. Take note if you have a narrow heel or high instep, for example, and select a shoe that will conform to the shape of your foot.

- If you wear orthotics, remember to bring them with you when you try on new shoes.

- Always try on shoes in the afternoon, because feet tend to swell during the day.

- Measure both feet, as many people find (to their surprise) that they have two different sizes.

- Have your feet re-measured from time to time, as their shape often changes over time, tending to elongate and widen over the years.

- If the shoes are not comfortable when you try them on in the store, don't buy them. You can't count on them stretching or "breaking in."

- Replace your shoes after 500 miles or so. Even if the sole shows no signs of wear, shock absorption properties can break down and affect your feet and joints.

—Courtesy of New Balance

The Clothes on Your Back

You will also need appropriate clothing. Once again, you can walk in any clothing, but for maximum benefit and comfort try to select clothes that are loose and can be worn in layers. The layer closest to your skin should be able to wick moisture away from your body as you work up a sweat. Remember that continuous walking, like all exercise, will elevate your core body temperature, so dress accordingly.

You may also want to buy a **heart rate monitor** or pedometer. Although certainly not required for walking, a heart rate monitor can help you make your walking workout more effective. Heart rate monitors tell you how fast your heart is beating during your workout and are a great way to gauge the intensity of your walk. The higher your heart rate (within your personalized zone) the more you are conditioning your heart. These devices usually come in the form of a wristwatch and a sensor that you wear across your chest. They vary in price from around thirty dollars for a basic monitor that will give you readouts of your heart rate, to in the hundreds for models with extra features such as providing the approximate number of calories you burned during your workout, and the amount of time you spent working within your target heart rate range. You can purchase a heart rate monitor at a sporting goods store or online. We will discuss the importance of heart rate in greater detail in the next chapter.

Pedometers are step counters. They record the number of steps that you take during your walk. Pedometers are appealing to people who prefer to view their walking progress in terms of steps rather than miles. You can also use pedometers to record the total number of steps you have walked throughout the day. This is not only fun to observe, it can make you realize how much—or how little—you walk in a given day. They are easy to wear, and clip to your waistband. Some pedometers also come with heart rate monitors built in. Whether you choose to use a pedometer, heart rate monitor, or both is largely a matter of personal preference.

Chapter 6
Gearing Up

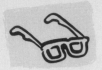

Walking with Mother Nature

If you choose to do your walking outside, you will need to know how to best approach environmental conditions that may affect the quality and safety of your workout. Here are some guidelines for common issues outdoor walkers face.

The Weather

In the cold. If you walk in the cold weather, you need to keep your body warm to prevent hypothermia, a dangerous (but easily preventable) condition that occurs when your internal body temperature drops below normal. To keep warm, it's a good idea to wear several layers of clothing in very cold temperatures. Warm air gets trapped between the layers to insulate your body. And whenever possible, it's best to dress in some of the new fabrics, such as polypro, which keep you dry even when wet.

Cotton isn't a good choice, because once wet (either from the weather or perspiration), it actually pulls warmth away from your body. Definitely wear a hat, as more than 50 percent of your body heat escapes through your head. Also, even though you may walk in freezing temperatures, the exercise will cause your body to sweat. In order to reduce the risk of significant heat loss, select clothing that traps air, but allows sweat to be wicked away from your body. Choose breathable fabrics such as polyester and cotton that allow your skin to air and your sweat to dry faster. Special microfiber materials are also available now that will pull the moisture away from your skin and up to the outer surface of the fabric. Avoid walking in heavy cotton sweats or material that is woven tightly because they will retain sweat and increase loss of body heat.

Ice and snow. Walking in winter comes with special considerations, such as how to best move through snow and ice. Insulated boots may be preferable in these conditions to keep your feet dry and warm. There are many options for winter footwear, so you may need to shop around a bit before you find the one that is best for you. A little snow or ice doesn't have to keep you from your daily walk. There are lots of ways to secure your footing. As always, it is a good idea to choose shoes appropriate for the climate and terrain you will be walking. A shoe with excellent traction is particularly important for the winter months when ice can form on the ground. Both snow and ice can be incredibly slippery underfoot. Boots or shoes with a good "grip" can help you keep your balance and avoid injury—not to mention some potential embarrassment. There are several products on the market designed to make walking on icy surfaces safe. YakTrax is one such product. This rubber traction device fits over your sneaker or boot; the metal coils on the bottom to give you good grip on ice and packed snow.

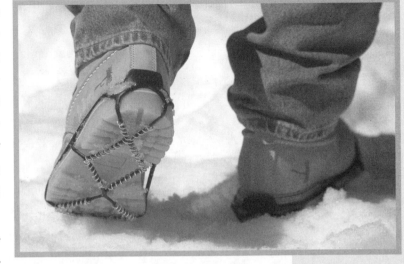

Wet. When it's wet and warm—more than 65 degrees or so—there's not much to worry about. Don't let the weather stop you. But wet in temperatures as high as 55 can lead to hypothermia.

When walking in hot weather, you want to prevent your body from overheating. The first line of defense when working out in hot, humid weather is to keep yourself hydrated in order to maintain your body temperature. Make sure that you drink 6 to 8 ounces of water every 15 to 20 minutes during your walk. Your clothing should be minimal in very hot weather to allow for better heat dissipation. Wear lightweight, loose fitting, light colored clothing. Cotton is a good choice during hot weather, because it absorbs water. Also use common sense. If the heat index is high, and we're in the middle of an ozone alert, take your walk indoors for the day in an air-conditioned environment like a shopping mall.

The sun. We all know how damaging exposure to the ultraviolet radiation of the sun's rays can be. But did you know that you need to protect yourself all year long from the sun's damaging effects, even in the dead of winter? The sun reflects off of cement and snow and exposes you to UV radiation when you least expect it. Whenever you walk outdoors, it's a good idea to wear sunglasses that offer UV protection, a hat, and of course sun block with a sun protection factor (SPF) of at least 15.

Treadmill Walking

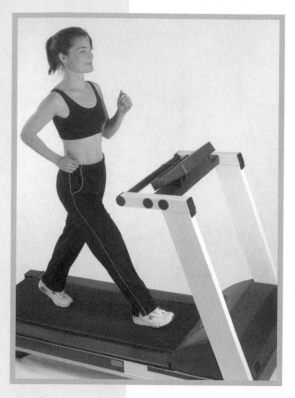

There is no denying that bad weather sometimes keeps us inside. It can be very hard to motivate yourself to go for a walk when it rains or snows, and going outside on particularly hot summer days is something that most of us don't get excited about. Walking indoors on a treadmill is a great option on days when the weather might otherwise keep us from exercising. Machines range from $300 to $3,000 and up, and have many different types of programming options. If you are thinking of buying a treadmill for use in your home, one very important consideration is its size. You may even want to take a tape measure with you to the sporting goods store. Make sure to test out different treadmills before you decide on a particular model. Several important factors to pay close attention to include the sturdiness of the machine and the smoothness of the ride—a belt that jerks instead of rolls is definitely unacceptable.

Safety Tips

You are enjoying your evening walk around your neighborhood, listening to your favorite music, dressed in your dark blue workout suit, when all of a sudden a car (that you didn't hear coming because you like your music loud) has to veer widely to the left and narrowly avoids hitting you (apparently you weren't visible because of your dark clothing). Though you might be shaken, you've just learned several important safety rules.

First, do not wear dark clothing when walking at night—it is important that you are visible. Wear light colored clothing as well as reflecting decals. In addition, do not use a personal headset stereo if it prevents you from hearing not only cars, but also a person who may be approaching (and who may be a potential threat). If you walk at night, select areas that are well-lit and where you are close to homes or businesses in case of an emergency (avoid parks and deserted areas).

Walking Staffs and Poles

A single walking staff or pair of poles can provide additional support and stability in particularly loose or uneven terrain. Poles and staffs can also help relieve stress on your ankles and knees, and are widely used by walkers with weak ankles, chronic injuries, and other problems like arthritis. Staffs and poles come in a variety of shapes and styles, for walking on both trails and urban streets. Some even have adjustable lengths that allow you to keep just the right angle for support when walking up and down hills. Others collapse for easy storage and can be very useful when you travel. A staff or pole may also provide some degree of security as a defense against potential attackers.

And if you come across barking dogs, don't panic. Many times, a dog will just bark at you and then leave. Never run when a dog approaches; it triggers the animal's chase instinct. Instead, slow down, avoiding eye contact with the dog, and continue on your way. Speaking firmly to the dog (Stay!) may help, too.

Chapter 7

Ready, Set, Go!

A re you ready to begin the *Walk the Weight Away!* Program; to put on your walking shoes and go? Sure you are. This eight-week program is progressive, meaning that it increases in intensity and level of challenge over time and includes the addition of a strength training program beginning in weeks two through four. By the end of the eight-week period, if you have followed both the walking program and the eating plan recommendations that we presented in Chapter 2, you will see a thinner, healthier you. Once you've finished the program, we are certain that walking will have become a habit, an activity that you truly enjoy and which you will continue for the rest of your life. Now, let's get down to the nitty gritty.

How to Walk

Proper posture is essential for fitness walking. In fact, it's a good idea to do a posture check in front of a mirror before you head out on your walk. Make sure your head is pulled back, that your back is straight, that your shoulders are down, that you have a natural arch in your spine, and that your weight is centered over your pelvis (many of us have a tendency to round our backs and shoulders and to push our heads forward beyond our necks). If you have poor posture, keeping your body in good form may feel awkward at first. Rest assured that over time it will become second nature, especially after you add strengthening exercises to your workout program. Remember to wear proper walking shoes and comfortable, loose clothing. As you walk, swing your arms naturally at your sides, breathe deeply, and walk with an energetic stride. And, don't forget to include your active warm up and post-walking stretches.

Intensity of Your Walk

There are three primary factors that determine the intensity of your walk: pace, terrain, and duration. Pace is the speed of your walk. Brisk walking—walking a mile in 15 minutes—is recommended for fitness benefits, because it is most likely to bring your heart rate into your training zone. However, many of you may be sedentary, and a 15-minute-mile may be too fast initially. That's why we begin with a pace of 20 minutes per mile during the first week in order to ease you into your walking program. As the weeks go by, you increase your pace and therefore increase the intensity of your workout. Remember, increasing the intensity will increase the number of calories you burn in each session, as well as the cardiovascular benefits of walking.

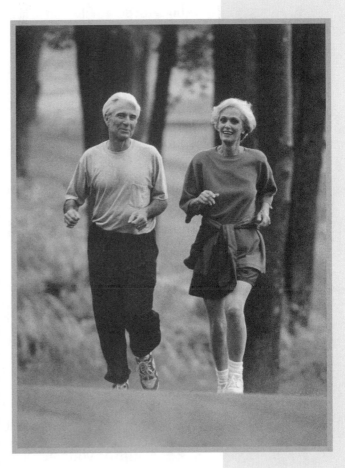

You may find you can increase your pace to the point where you are race-walking, which is a bit different from regular walking. We'll take a few minutes here to talk about this great form of exercise. Race-walking can give you the cardiovascular and calorie burning benefits of running without all that impact to your bones and limbs. Its pace is extremely fast (as fast as six miles an hour) and you are somewhere between walking and running—you are on the verge of a run, but you are still walking. Form for race-walking is different than for fitness walking. In a race-walk your heel should hit the ground with each step and roll forward just as your other heel is lifted. Your arms swing fast and your hips move forward and back in order to maintain your pace. Maintaining a fast pace without breaking into a run requires a great deal of control and contraction of muscles in the legs and abdominals. It is tough and only for the very advanced walker who wants to take his or her walking program to the next level.

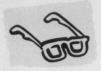

Walking up and down hills leads to shapely legs!

Terrain or grade is another factor that greatly determines the intensity of your walk. It refers to how flat or hilly a surface is. Flat ground is easier to walk on; we can walk much faster on flat ground than on hills. By gradually adding some hills to your walk you make your heart work much harder as your leg muscles have to contract with greater force in order to pull your body over a hill. That adds to greater effort, and therefore, increases the intensity of your walk. It also provides a great toning exercise for your legs.

In addition to pace and terrain, distance or duration will determine how many calories you burn. Simply put, the greater distance you walk at a given pace, the more calories you will burn because you are working out for a longer period of time. You will begin your walking program with a 30-minute walk and then we will increase the distance.

Ready to Go

Here's all you need to do to begin your *Walk the Weight Away!* Program.

- Determine your weight-loss goals (remember, be realistic and aim for a weight loss of no more than 2 pounds per week.)

- Review the nutrition section and study the food pyramid.

- Walk at least three times each week for at least 30 minutes each session—five is best for weight loss and health benefits.

- Monitor your heart rate to make sure you are working at the proper intensity for weight loss and health benefits.

- Record your eating and walking habits in the diary pages in Part II.

- Enjoy your walk and your new, healthier way of living!

Walk the **Weight Away!**

Outline of the *Walk the Weight Away!* Program

In the workbook section that follows you will find eight weeks worth of program record pages. On the left-hand page is your food diary; on the right-hand page is your workout diary. Use these pages to record and monitor your progress. Your goal is to walk a minimum of three times a week. Ideally, and especially if you are trying to lose weight, you want to walk at least five times a week. Here are the phases for your *Walk the Weight Away!* Program.

Phase I: First Steps. In Week 1 you're taking your first steps. Here you must gauge your starting point. Determine what is realistic for you, given your current level of activity. If you hardly ever walk unless you have to, begin at the 20-minute per mile pace (or even slower if need be). You want to feel that your walk gives you a workout—you should feel a slight sweat, and your heart rate should increase into the lower end of your training zone (review the information on heart rates in chapter 5). You should never walk so fast that you are out of breath, or unable to talk. **During Week One you ease into the program and do only a few stretches, walk three days and don't do strength training.**

Phase II: Commitment. In weeks two through four you are in the commitment phase of the program. **During this time you increase the distance or time of each walking session. You will also begin strength training sessions three times each week.**

Phase III: Results. Now you are really on track to up the intensity and shed even more fat. In weeks five through eight you will increase your pace and even add hills if you'd like to turn the heat up on calorie burning.

You can keep track of your walking by the time you spend walking (or the miles you walk). You also alternatively can count the number of steps you walk, which requires the purchase of a pedometer. Whichever method best motivates you is the one to choose.

Get a Buddy, Get a Group

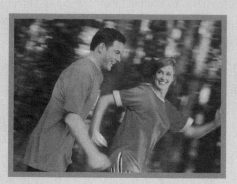

There are many wonderful reasons to walk alone. You can listen to your favorite songs, meditate, take in the sights and sounds of nature, and really focus on your breathing and on the intensity of your workout. Many people, however, prefer to walk with someone else, or to walk as part of a group. If you think you are one of those people, a walking club may be right for you.

Why a Club?

Walking with a group of people can make you forget that you are exercising. In fact, many studies have shown that people tend to stick to an exercise routine if they work out with a friend. As you talk to your fellow walkers you will find that the time just flies by and, before you know it, you've reached the end of your route. Your walk will feel as much a social outing as an exercise session.

In addition to preventing boredom, walking with others can increase motivation. If you know that your fellow walkers are counting on you to be there, you will be more apt to walk—even on those low-energy days when you might otherwise blow off your walk if you were walking alone. Club members can challenge each other to walk a little faster, or a little farther, and encourage each other along the way. A club also provides an instant reward system. You can give each other awards for distance achieved or create special tee-shirts with your club's name and logo.

Walk
the
Weight
Away!

Kinds of Clubs

A walking club can be as informal as getting a couple of friends together on a regular basis. Each member can take turns plotting out the route for the day, varying the intensity in order to keep the walks interesting. An informal club comprised of friends with similar fitness goals is also a great way to keep in touch with your friends—if you are like many busy people, carving out social time can be difficult. With your walking club you not only see and talk to friends, you get your workout in at the same time.

Another option is to join a formal walking club in your area. The International Volkssport Association (IVV), the largest association of walking clubs, is a good place to start researching clubs in your town or city. Its United States branch, The American Volkssport Association is comprised of 350 national walking clubs, which organize 3000 walking events each year. Check out its Web site, www.ava.org, for more information on clubs and walking events. You can also inquire at health clubs, local papers, local recreation centers, walking magazines, and sports stores for other local walking clubs.

If your area does not already have a walking club, you may want to start one of your own. Bear in mind that clubs connected to a school or other existing non-profit organization do not need to be incorporated. But if your club will have its own financial accounts, you will need to get a tax ID and incorporate.

You can advertise for members by placing flyers up at local sports stores, schools, churches, community centers, malls, and health clubs. You also can run an ad in your local paper. Word of mouth also works well for these types of club.

Whether you decide to join an informal or formal walking club, the camaraderie and energy you receive from participating in a common activity with a group of people is a great source of motivation.

Tracking Your Progress

For each day that you walk, fill in a workbook page. We offer three ways for you to record your walking workout:

- distance walked
- time walked
- steps taken (for this option you need a pedometer)

If your workout for that day differed from our suggestion, just cross out our suggestions and write in what you did instead. For example, some days, you may feel extra energetic and decide you want to walk for an hour when we have suggested that you walk for a half hour. That's great. Other days, you may not feel so well and may have to walk a bit slower than our recommendation. No problem. That's why you have these diary pages, to tailor the program to your needs and to use the record as a way to gauge your progress and what you need to work on.

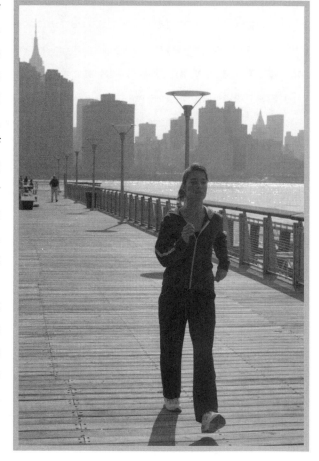

Each day (regardless of whether or not you walk) you should also fill in your food diary page, indicating when you ate, with whom, and how you felt about what you ate.

Most important, don't forget to set goals for the next day and to read the inspirational quotes to keep your motivation high.

Part 2

Walk the Weight Away!, Day-by-Day

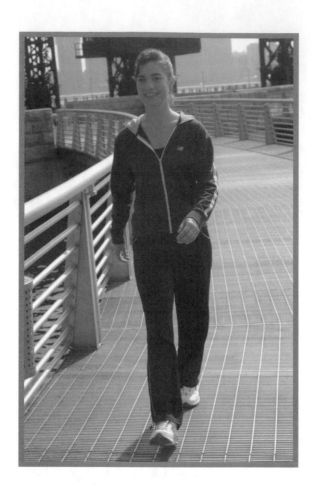

Walk the Weight Away! Workbook Pages

Welcome to your *Walk the Weight Away!* Workbook. Each day gets two pages: One is your Nutrition Guide and the other is your Workout Journal.

Each **Nutrition Guide** page includes menu suggestions and a place to record what you ate that day. There's a spot to check off how many glasses of water you drank. You'll also find a place to record how you felt about that day's food choices. Don't think of this as a report card, but rather a way to track your eating patterns. We also ask you to set a goal for the next day's meals: Maybe you'd like to drink more water or try skipping your afternoon soda.

A Word About Measurements

Measuring everything you eat gets tedious. That's why our recipes use fast and easy measurements:

1 plate, 1/2 plate, or 1/4 plate. We're talking about portions of a standard size dinner plate.

Bowl. When we say "a bowl of," we mean a cereal/soup bowl three-quarters full.

Cup. A coffee mug.

Handful. Small handful of the food; there shouldn't be any hanging out between your fingers.

Heaping teaspoon/tablespoon. Use the spoons in your silverware drawer, not measuring spoons.

Small plate. A standard dessert/salad plate.

Each **Workout Journal** page guides you through the day's activities, from walking and weight training to stretching. Each day you'll stretch (after warming up) and most days you'll walk. On "rest" days (that is, days you don't walk), we offer helpful tips to make your workouts more enjoyable and more effective.

In the **First Steps Phase** (week one), you'll stretch every day, and walk three days to help you ease into the program.

In the **Commitment Phase** (weeks two through four), you'll walk four or five days a week, picking up the pace and gradually increasing distance. You'll also add weight training to the mix. Although you'll find weight training options on five days each week, aim to lift weights three days. This may be the most important phase of the program, since it's when you'll be turning walking into a habit.

In the **Results Phase** (weeks five through eight), we crank it up another notch with added distance and increased time. You'll be burning lots of fat, too. Here's where you'll really start to notice changes in how you look and feel.

Nutrition Guide

Suggested Menu

Breakfast

2 packets instant oatmeal

1 small box raisins

1 cup non-fat milk

Lunch

• Veggie Pita Sandwich
(page 59)

1 apple

1 handful nuts

Dinner

• 1 piece Crispy Chicken
(page 69)

• ¼ plate Smashed Potatoes
(page 89)

½ plate steamed
green beans

1 individual container
applesauce

Snacks

1 large handful grapes

152

Your goal this week is to pay attention to what and how you eat.

On every day of this program, you'll find menu suggestions for three meals and one snack. Feel free to substitute any of the other meal or snack ideas on pages 46 to 92.

Fill out the food diary each day. At week's end, make note of any patterns that emerge. Do you tend to eat when you're angry? Bored? Happy? Sad? Once you identify those patterns, you can begin to make different choices.

August 23rd 2009

Breakfast time: 9 am

What I ate _chinese sweet bread_
glass of OJ

What I was doing while I ate
sitting down w/ kogyi

Hunger level _not hungry_

Lunch time: 12:30

What I ate _____

What I was doing while I ate
sitting down w/ kogyi

Hunger level _VERY !_

Dinner time: 8:30 pm

What I ate _____

What I was doing while I ate
cooking & sitting down w/ kogyi

Hunger level _∅_

Snack after dinner time:

What I ate _pineapple_

What I was doing while I ate
_____

Hunger level _∅_

Water

Remember to drink 8 glasses of water

I feel __ about how I ate today:

☒ satisfied

☐ proud

☐ disappointed

☐ other _____

My goals for tomorrow:

_____

_____

_____

Walk
the
Weight
Away!

Workout Journal

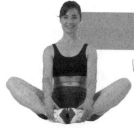

Pre-Walk Warm-Up

☐ **Spend 5 to 10 minutes slowly getting ready for your workout.**

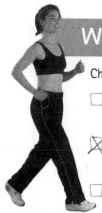

Walking Workout

Choose one.

☐ **Distance: 1.5 miles**
(20-minute-per-mile pace)

☒ **Time: 30 min.**
(20-minute-per-mile pace)

☐ **Steps: 3000 steps**

3.3 mph
≈ 18 minute/mile pace

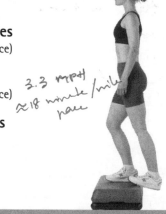

Post-Walk Stretches

☐ **Neck Stretch,** page 107
☐ **Hamstring Stretch,** page 114
☐ **Quadriceps Stretch,** page 113
☐ **Calf Stretch,** page 115

Quote of the Day
A journey of a thousand miles must begin with a single step.
—Chinese proverb

Trainer's Tip
Take a photograph of yourself today, the first day of your journey to better health. Then on the last day of the program, take another to record your success. Glue both pictures in the spaces provided on page 265.

153

I feel __ about my workout today:
☐ satisfied
☐ proud
☐ disappointed
☐ other _____

My goals for tomorrow:
_____
_____
_____

Part 2
Walk the Weight Away!,
Day by Day

Nutrition Guide

Suggested Menu

Breakfast

- 3 Whole Wheat Pancakes with Strawberry Syrup (page 54, page 53)

  1 cup non-fat milk

Lunch

- Heart-Healthy Egg Salad Sandwich (page 56)

  1 raw cucumber sliced

  1 apple

Dinner

- 1 portion Southwestern Pork Tenderloin (page 77)

  1 ear corn

  ½ plate mixed vegetable salad

  1 tablespoon low-fat salad dressing

Snacks

1 cup juice

154

Walk the **Weight** **Away!**

If you didn't find yesterday's menu items filling, try these strategies:

- Drink a large glass of water about 10 minutes before eating. You'll feel fuller and eat less.
- Prepare a relaxing environment for you and your family as you eat.
- Take your time—don't wolf down your food! When you eat more slowly, you'll be more aware of how the food smells and tastes.
- Before reaching for second helpings, wait 10 minutes. You'll often find that you're satisfied after all.

August 24, 2005

Breakfast   time:

What I ate _toast + butter + strawberry jam + OJ_

What I was doing while I ate _sitting w/ kiggi_

Hunger level ___2___

Lunch   time:

What I ate _salad_

What I was doing while I ate _sitting @ work_

Hunger level ___1___

Dinner   time:

What I ate _soup_

What I was doing while I ate

Hunger level ___0___

Snack   time:

What I ate _dried apples_

What I was doing while I ate _working 3-4 pm_

Hunger level ___3___

Water

Remember to drink 8 glasses of water

I feel ___ about how I ate today:

- [ ] satisfied
- [ ] proud
- [ ] disappointed
- [ ] other _____

My goals for tomorrow:

_____

_____

_____

Workout Journal

Daily Stretches

☐ Head & Neck Stretch, page 107   ☐ The Egg, page 112
☐ Shoulder Stretch, page 108   ☐ Quadriceps Stretch, page 113
☐ Triceps Stretch, page 109   ☐ Hamstring Stretch, page 114
☐ Chest & Biceps Stretch, page 110   ☐ Calf Stretch, page 115
☐ Upper Back Stretch, page 111

Map Your Way Across the USA

When you're starting a new journey toward fitness, it's inspiring to track your progress. Here's one way to keep track of how far you'll be walking in the weeks and months to come. All it takes is a map of the United States, some stick pins, and a magic marker. Place a stick pin in the map where you're starting—your hometown, for instance. Then, choose an ending point—maybe a town or site across the country. Place a stick pin there, too. Then, as your miles add up, trace your progress across the map with a magic marker. For instance, let's say that after following your walking program for 1 week, you've covered 5 miles. That may take you to the next town, so draw a line. Keep tracking your progress until you cross the country—it's a wonderful motivator.

Warm-Up

You're not scheduled to walk today, but you still need to warm up before you do your stretches. A good time to do them is the late afternoon, after you've been up and around all day—you're more likely to be loose.

Fit Tips

Since you're going slowly during the first steps phase, it's the perfect time to practice your form. Here are some tips to keep in mind.

① Stand straight and tall.

② Keep your head up.

③ Don't squeeze your hands into a fist; keep them relaxed.

④ Keep your shoulders back and relaxed.

Quote of the Day
Goals that are not written down are just wishes.
—Anonymous

.2 miles
@ 3.3 MPH.
5 min warmup
30 min 3.3 - 3.5 MPH

155

Part 2
Walk the Weight Away!,
Day by Day

Nutrition Guide

Suggested Menu

Breakfast

- Strawberry Orange Muffin (page 52)

  1 banana

  1 cup non-fat milk

Lunch

- Updated Sloppy Joe Sandwich (page 58)

  1 orange

Dinner

- ¼ plate Teriyaki Steak Fingers (page 81)
- ¼ plate Smashed Potatoes (page 89)

  1 small vegetable salad

  2 shakes low-fat salad dressing

Snacks

1 small container no-sugar added yogurt

156

Walk the **Weight** Away!

You've been watching what you eat, but what about what you drink? You'd be surprised by how quickly calories in beverages can add up.

That extra 610 calories a day is enough to sabotage your weight-loss efforts. You don't need to give up your favorite beverage, just be mindful of how many extra calories each adds.

Beverage	No. of Calories
Coffee, with 2 tablespoons half and-half and 2 teaspoons sugar	160
8 ounces orange juice	110
1 12-ounce can soda	140
1 8-ounce bottle iced tea	200
Total	610

August 26, 2009

Breakfast   time:

What I ate _toast + jam + butter_

_OJ_

What I was doing while I ate

sitting down wt kogyi

Hunger level _1_

Lunch   time:

What I ate _soup + hf-oust:_

What I was doing while I ate

@ work

Hunger level _____

Dinner   time:

What I ate _soup_

What I was doing while I ate

sitting down wt kogyi

Hunger level _2._

Snack   time:

What I ate _ice cream_

What I was doing while I ate

@ work around 4.

Hunger level _____

Water

Remember to drink 8 glasses of water

I feel ___ about how I ate today:

- [ ] satisfied
- [ ] proud
- [ ] disappointed
- [ ] other _____

My goals for tomorrow:

_____

_____

Workout Journal

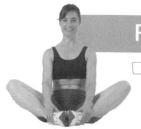

Pre-Walk Warm-Up

☐ **Spend 5 to 10 minutes slowly swinging your arms to prepare for your workout.**

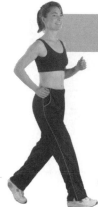

Walking Workout

Choose one.

☐ **Distance: 1.5 miles**
(20-minute-per-mile pace)

☒ **Time: 30 min.**
(20-minute-per-mile pace)

☐ **Steps: 3000 steps**

2.3 – 3.4 mph
2 miles.
≈ 180 kcal burned

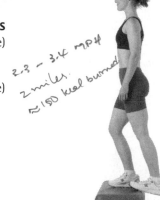

Post-Walk Stretches

☐ **Neck Stretch,** page 107
☐ **Hamstring Stretch,** page 114
☐ **Quadriceps Stretch,** page 113
☐ **Calf Stretch,** page 115

I feel ___ about my workout today:

☐ satisfied
☐ proud
☐ disappointed
☐ other _____

My goals for tomorrow:

_____

_____

_____

Quote of the Day
Walking is the best possible exercise. Habituate yourself to walk very far.
—Thomas Jefferson

Trainer's Tip
Enjoy your walk. Look around, take in everything around you; breathe deeply to bring oxygen to your working muscles.

157

Part 2
Walk the Weight Away!, Day by Day

Nutrition Guide

Suggested Menu

Breakfast

3 frozen pancakes topped with 2 heaping tablespoons warmed applesauce

1 cup non-fat milk

Lunch

- 2 slices Pizza Primavera (page 73)

1 handful pretzels

Dinner

1 low-fat hotdog

1 hotdog roll

1 handful low-fat chips

¼ plate baked beans

Snack

½ bag light microwave pop-corn

Are you a life-long member of the clean plate club? Maybe it's time to give up your membership. Finishing everything on your plate just because it's there isn't necessarily a healthy way to eat. In restaurants, where portions tend to be gargantuan, you should consider eating only half the food and saving the rest for the following day's lunch. When at home, serve yourself small portions that you know you can finish without feeling stuffed.

Breakfast   time:

What I ate _____

_____

What I was doing while I ate

_____

Hunger level _____

Lunch   time:

What I ate _____

_____

What I was doing while I ate

_____

Hunger level _____

Dinner   time:

What I ate _____

_____

What I was doing while I ate

_____

Hunger level _____

Snack   time:

What I ate _____

_____

What I was doing while I ate

_____

Hunger level _____

Water

Remember to drink 8 glasses of water

I feel ___ about how I ate today:

- ☐ satisfied
- ☐ proud
- ☐ disappointed
- ☐ other _____

My goals for tomorrow:

_____

_____

_____

158

Walk the **Weight Away!**

Workout Journal

Daily Stretches

- [ ] Head & Neck Stretch, page 107
- [ ] Shoulder Stretch, page 108
- [ ] Triceps Stretch, page 109
- [ ] Chest & Biceps Stretch, page 110
- [ ] Upper Back Stretch, page 111
- [ ] The Egg, page 112
- [ ] Quadriceps Stretch, page 113
- [ ] Hamstring Stretch, page 114
- [ ] Calf Stretch, page 115
- [ ] Butterfly Stretch, page 116

A Family Affair

Getting your family involved in your walking program may make it more enjoyable. Here are some ways to make it appealing to the younger set.

1. Plan for a (non-food) treat at the end of the walk.
2. Make a game of sighting cars, dogs, or birds.
3. Stop by your children's friends' homes and pick them up for the walk—turn it into a parade.
4. Older children may enjoy spending special time with parents.

Quote of the Day

It's choice—not chance—that determines your destiny.
—Jean Nidetch

159

Part 2
Walk the Weight Away!,
Day by Day

Nutrition Guide

Suggested Menu

Breakfast

- 1 Spinach Salad (page 46)
  1 small banana
  1 cup non-fat milk

Lunch

- 1 ½ cups Thai Pasta Salad
  (page 91)
  1 pear

Dinner

- 1 bowl Pasta Primavera
  (page 72)
  1 small vegetable salad
  2 shakes low-fat
  salad dressing
  1 slice Italian bread

Snack

1 handful baked tortillas
with salsa

When you're trying to lose weight, B-U-F-F-E-T can spell trouble. How can you not overeat when you're faced with a huge expanse of food? Start with a plan. Before you pick up your plate, take a *slow* stroll along the tables, making careful choices about the foods you want. That walk will help you be more mindful, which just might be enough to help you avoid a feeding frenzy.

Breakfast   time:

What I ate _____

_____

What I was doing while I ate

_____

Hunger level _____

Lunch   time:

What I ate _____

_____

What I was doing while I ate

_____

Hunger level _____

Dinner   time:

What I ate _____

_____

What I was doing while I ate

_____

Hunger level _____

Snack   time:

What I ate _____

_____

What I was doing while I ate

_____

Hunger level _____

Water

Remember to drink 8 glasses of water

I feel ___ about how I ate today:

- ☐ satisfied
- ☐ proud
- ☐ disappointed
- ☐ other _____

My goals for tomorrow:

_____

_____

_____

Walk the Weight Away!

Workout Journal

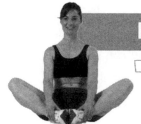

Pre-Walk Warm-Up

☐ **Spend 5 to 10 minutes slowly swinging your arms to prepare for your workout.**

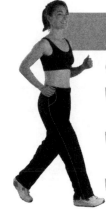

Walking Workout

Choose one.

☐ **Distance: 1.5 miles**
(20-minute-per-mile pace)

☐ **Time: 30 min.**
(20-minute-per-mile pace)

☐ **Steps: 3000 steps**

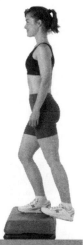

Post-Walk Stretches

☐ **Neck Stretch,** page 107
☐ **Hamstring Stretch,** page 114
☐ **Quadriceps Stretch,** page 113
☐ **Calf Stretch,** page 115

Quote of the Day

Most people never run far enough on their first wind to find out if they've got a second. Give your dreams all you've got and you'll be amazed at the energy that comes out of you.
—William James

Trainer's Tip

If you feel any pain when stretching, ease up on the stretch. Avoid stretching so deeply that your muscles start to shake; this is a sign of over-stretching and can lead to injury.

161

Part 2
Walk the Weight Away!,
Day by Day

I feel __ about my workout today:

☐ satisfied
☐ proud
☐ disappointed
☐ other _____

My goals for tomorrow:

_____
_____
_____

Nutrition Guide

Suggested Menu

Breakfast

- 2 slices French Toast
  (page 49)

  1 orange

  1 slice Canadian bacon

Lunch

- 1 Strawberry Orange
  Muffin (page 52)

  1 apple

  1 small container non-fat,
  no sugar added yogurt

Dinner

- ¼ plate Spaghetti Squash
  Pomodoro (page 78)

  ¼ plate vegetable salad

  1 cup strawberries

Snack

1 slice string cheese with
3 crackers

162

Walk
the
Weight
Away!

From the time we're children, we learn to associate food with treats and rewards: We get a cookie for an A on a report card and an ice cream cone for behaving well at the shopping mall. As adults we treat ourselves with big fruity cocktails or a chocolate bar for getting through a long work week. If you tend to reward yourself with high-calorie foods, try treating yourself with non-food rewards: a manicure, tickets to a ball game, or a visit to a friend.

Breakfast	time:

What I ate _____

_____

What I was doing while I ate

_____

Hunger level _____

Lunch	time:

What I ate _____

_____

What I was doing while I ate

_____

Hunger level _____

Dinner	time:

What I ate _____

_____

What I was doing while I ate

_____

Hunger level _____

Snack	time:

What I ate _____

_____

What I was doing while I ate

_____

Hunger level _____

Water ⊔⊔⊔⊔⊔⊔⊔⊔

Remember to drink 8 glasses of water

I feel ___ about how I ate today:

☐ satisfied

☐ proud

☐ disappointed

☐ other _____

My goals for tomorrow:

_____

_____

_____

Workout Journal

Daily Stretches

- [ ] Head & Neck Stretch, page 107
- [ ] Shoulder Stretch, page 108
- [ ] Triceps Stretch, page 109
- [ ] Chest & Biceps Stretch, page 110
- [ ] Upper Back Stretch, page 111
- [ ] The Egg, page 112
- [ ] Quadriceps Stretch, page 113
- [ ] Hamstring Stretch, page 114
- [ ] Calf Stretch, page 115
- [ ] Butterfly Stretch, page 116

It's Not All or Nothing

Remember, if you've been sedentary for a long, it's important to respect your limits. If you're not able to walk for 20 minutes (or 1.5 miles or 3000 steps) straight, don't. Walk in 5- to 10-minute increments throughout the day until you're able to walk for the full 20 minutes. Not only will you reap many of the same benefits, but you're less likely to become discouraged—and that will increase your chances of success.

Leave the Weights at Home

You may have seen people walking wearing ankle weights. That's not a good idea, especially for beginners. Ankle weights can stress your hip and knee joints.

Take Your Act on the Road

Vacation time coming up? That's no reason to let your walking program slide. Almost every vacation affords opportunity for walking: Go sight-seeing or window shopping for a day; take walks on the beach. Every step counts!

Quote of the Day
Even if you're on the right track, you'll get run over if you just sit there.
—Will Rogers

163

Part 2
Walk the Weight Away!,
Day by Day

Nutrition Guide

Suggested Menu

Breakfast

1 bowl high-fiber cereal

1 cup non-fat milk

1 handful nuts

Lunch

- 1 cup Cheese Ravioli Soup (page 63)

4 saltines

1 apple

Dinner

- 1 piece Buttery Almond Fish (page 62)

¼ plate brown rice

½ plate broccoli

1 cup non-fat milk

Snack

1 cup fresh berries

You've reached the end of Week 1—did you fill out your food and workout diary each day? Can you identify any patterns about your eating habits? Use what you've learned not to punish yourself, but to make more informed choices about how you eat.

SEPT. 2

Breakfast   time:

What I ate _____

_____

What I was doing while I ate

_____

Hunger level _____

Lunch   time:

What I ate _____

_____

What I was doing while I ate

_____

Hunger level _____

Dinner   time:

What I ate _____

_____

What I was doing while I ate

_____

Hunger level _____

Snack   time:

What I ate _____

_____

What I was doing while I ate

_____

Hunger level _____

Water

Remember to drink 8 glasses of water

I feel ___ about how I ate today:

☐ satisfied

☐ proud

☐ disappointed

☐ other _____

My goals for tomorrow:

_____

_____

_____

Walk the **Weight** Away!

Workout Journal

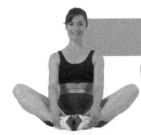

Pre-Walk Warm-Up

☐ **Spend 5 to 10 minutes slowly swinging your arms to prepare for your workout.**

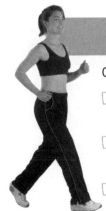

Walking Workout

Choose one.

☐ **Distance: 1.5 miles**
(20-minute-per-mile pace)

☐ **Time: 30 min.**
(20-minute-per-mile pace)

☐ **Steps: 3000 steps**

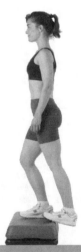

Post-Walk Stretches

☐ **Neck Stretch,** page 107
☐ **Hamstring Stretch,** page 114
☐ **Quadriceps Stretch,** page 113
☐ **Calf Stretch,** page 115

Quote of the Day
The harder you work, the luckier you get.
—Unknown

Trainer's Tip
On especially warm days, you may want to bring a small bottle of water along with you on your walks. But skip the sports drinks you see advertised on television. They're designed to replace electrolytes, which your body loses after about an hour of very intense exercise; for workouts that last less than an hour they simply add calories.

165

I feel __ about my workout today:
☐ satisfied
☐ proud
☐ disappointed
☐ other _____

My goals for tomorrow:
_____
_____
_____

Part 2
Walk the Weight Away!, Day by Day

Nutrition Guide

Suggested Menu

Breakfast

½ large bagel

2 heaping teaspoons peanut butter

1 small box raisins

1 cup non-fat milk

Lunch

• Lemon Hummus Sandwich (page 57)

1 orange

Dinner

½ plate baked ham

¼ plate brown rice

• ¼ plate Cheesy Broccoli Gratin (page 83)

1 kiwifruit

Snack

2 large graham crackers

To weigh or not to weigh—that is the question. Oftentimes, when people start a weight-loss program, they jump on the scale each morning eager to see results. Trouble is, your weight can fluxuate by as much as a few pounds from day to day—mostly due to changes in the amount of water in your body. Seeing a weight gain after three days of dieting can be very discouraging. That's why experts recommend stepping on the scale once a week at most.

Breakfast time:
What I ate _____
_____
What I was doing while I ate
_____
Hunger level _____

Lunch time:
What I ate _____
_____
What I was doing while I ate
_____
Hunger level _____

Dinner time:
What I ate _____
_____
What I was doing while I ate
_____
Hunger level _____

Snack time:
What I ate _____
_____
What I was doing while I ate
_____
Hunger level _____

Water

Remember to drink 8 glasses of water

I feel ___ about how I ate today:

☐ satisfied

☐ proud

☐ disappointed

☐ other _____

My goals for tomorrow:

_____

_____

_____

166

Walk
the
Weight
Away!

Workout Journal

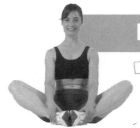

Pre-Walk Warm-Up

☐ **Spend 5 to 10 minutes slowly swinging your arms to prepare for your workout.**

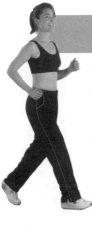

Walking Workout

Choose one.

☐ **Distance: 2 miles**
(15-minute-per-mile pace)

☐ **Time: 30 min.**
(15-minute-per-mile pace)

☐ **Steps: 4000 steps**

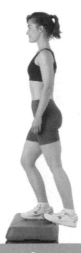

Strength Training

(1 set of 10 to 15 repetitions)

☐ **Shoulders Up,** page 118
☐ **Arm Power I,** page 119
☐ **Front Fly,** page 125
☐ **Back Fly,** page 122
☐ **Thigh Shaper,** page 126
☐ **Best Butt,** page 127
☐ **Six Pack,** page 132
☐ **Basic Crunch,** page 133

Post-Walk Stretches

☐ **Neck Stretch,** page 107
☐ **Shoulder Stretch,** page 108
☐ **Upper Back Stretch,** page 111
☐ **Hamstring Stretch,** page 114
☐ **Quad Stretch,** page 113
☐ **Calf Stretch,** page 115

I feel __ about my workout today:

☐ satisfied
☐ proud
☐ disappointed
☐ other _____

My goals for tomorrow:

_____

_____

_____

Quote of the Day
Obstacles are those frightful things you see when you take your eyes off your goal.
—Henry Ford

Trainer's Tip
When you lift weights, always exhale during the exertion phase of the exercise (when you are working against gravity to lift the weight).

167

Part 2
Walk the Weight Away!,
Day by Day

Nutrition Guide

Psychologists tell us that it takes about 21 days to break a habit or build a new one. That's what the Commitment Phase is all about. Over the next three weeks you'll slowly incorporate new habits into your daily routine. Before you know it, making healthy choices will come naturally.

Suggested Menu

Breakfast
- 1 Graham Cracker Muffin (page 50)

  1 cup non-fat milk

  1 small banana

Lunch
- 1 bowl Stovetop Lentil Casserole (page 80)

  4 saltines

  1 plum

Dinner
- 1 piece Grilled Marinated Salmon (page 70)
- ¼ plate Rice Pilaf (page 87)
- ½ plate Spinach Salad (page 90)

Snack
½ baked potato with salsa

168

Walk the Weight Away!

Breakfast	time:

What I ate _____

_____

What I was doing while I ate

_____

Hunger level _____

Lunch	time:

What I ate _____

_____

What I was doing while I ate

_____

Hunger level _____

Dinner	time:

What I ate _____

_____

What I was doing while I ate

_____

Hunger level _____

Snack	time:

What I ate _____

_____

What I was doing while I ate

_____

Hunger level _____

Water ▯▯▯▯▯▯▯▯▯▯
Remember to drink 8 glasses of water

I feel ___ about how I ate today:
- ☐ satisfied
- ☐ proud
- ☐ disappointed
- ☐ other _____

My goals for tomorrow:

_____

_____

_____

Workout Journal

Daily Stretches

- ☐ Head & Neck Stretch, page 107
- ☐ Shoulder Stretch, page 108
- ☐ Triceps Stretch, page 109
- ☐ Chest & Biceps Stretch, page 110
- ☐ Upper Back Stretch, page 111

- ☐ The Egg, page 112
- ☐ Quadriceps Stretch, page 113
- ☐ Hamstring Stretch, page 114
- ☐ Calf Stretch, page 115
- ☐ Butterfly Stretch, page 116

Walk Softly

Shin splints are a painful condition that many people experience when they start walking or jogging. The good news is that there are several ways to avoid the condition:

❶ Always warm up well before you walk.

❷ Stick to soft surfaces whenever possible: grassy or dirt paths are good; asphalt is easier on the legs than concrete.

❸ Avoid abrupt changes in either your speed or terrain. If you've been walking slowly for a week, don't suddenly speed up. Likewise, if you're used to walking on grass, don't suddenly switch to concrete.

❹ Stretch well after walking.

Say No to Cotton Socks

Yes, clean, white cotton socks look great and feel good—initially—but they're not a good choice for fitness walking. Because cotton absorbs perspiration from your feet and traps it, and that can lead to painful rubbing and blisters. Stick to synthetic materials such as polypro.

Quote of the Day
Motivation is what gets you started. Habit is what keeps you going.
—Jim Ryun

169

Part 2
Walk the Weight Away!,
Day by Day

Nutrition Guide

Suggested Menu

Breakfast
- Greek Omelette (page 51)
  - ½ English muffin
  - 1 teaspoon jam
  - 1 cup berries

Lunch
- 1 plate vegetable salad
- 1 handful grapes
- ½ small whole grain bagel
- 1 teaspoon butter

Dinner
- ¾ cup Barbecued Pork (page 61)
- 1 whole grain hamburger bun
- 1 cup vegetable salad
- 1 small watermelon wedge

Snack
- 1 Strawberry Orange Muffin (page 52)

170

Walk the Weight Away!

Fall off the diet wagon? Maybe you had extra helpings and dessert at a special dinner. Don't worry: Overeating one day does *not* negate all your hard work. The trick is not to let one disappointing day discourage you into returning to old habits.

Breakfast   time:

What I ate _____

_____

What I was doing while I ate

_____

Hunger level _____

Lunch   time:

What I ate _____

_____

What I was doing while I ate

_____

Hunger level _____

Dinner   time:

What I ate _____

_____

What I was doing while I ate

_____

Hunger level _____

Snack   time:

What I ate _____

_____

What I was doing while I ate

_____

Hunger level _____

Water

Remember to drink 8 glasses of water

I feel __ about how I ate today:
- ☐ satisfied
- ☐ proud
- ☐ disappointed
- ☐ other _____

My goals for tomorrow:

_____

_____

_____

Workout Journal

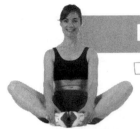

Pre-Walk Warm-Up

☐ **Spend 5 to 10 minutes slowly swinging your arms to prepare for your workout.**

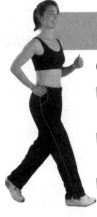

Walking Workout

Choose one.

☐ **Distance: 2 miles**
(15-minute-per-mile pace)

☐ **Time: 30 min.**
(15-minute-per-mile pace)

☐ **Steps: 4000 steps**

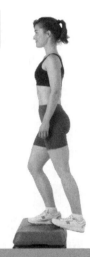

Strength Training

(1 set of 10 to 15 repetitions)
☐ **Arm Power II,** page 120
☐ **Tri Blaster,** page 121
☐ **Karate Kick,** page 128
☐ **Plié Press,** page 129
☐ **Hot Calves,** page 130
☐ **Strong Center,** page 131
☐ **Crunch Combo,** page 134

Post-Walk Stretches

☐ **Neck Stretch,** page 107
☐ **Chest & Biceps Stretch,** page 110
☐ **Triceps Stretch,** page 109
☐ **Hamstring Stretch,** page 114
☐ **Quad Stretch,** page 113
☐ **Calf Stretch,** page 115

I feel __ about my workout today:
☐ satisfied
☐ proud
☐ disappointed
☐ other _____

My goals for tomorrow:

_____

_____

_____

Quote of the Day
I can feel guilty about the past, apprehensive about the future, but only in the present can I act.
—Abraham Maslow

Trainer's Tip
Never lift a weight that's so heavy you begin to compensate by leaning back or losing form in some other way. Good form is essential for success and safety.

171

Part 2
Walk the Weight Away!,
Day by Day

Nutrition Guide

Suggested Menu

Breakfast

2 slices whole-grain toast

2 teaspoons jam

½ pint scrambled egg substitute, scrambled

½ grapefruit

Lunch

• 1 cup Chunky Beef & Vegetable Soup (page 67)

½ bagel

1 teaspoon butter

Dinner

• 1 bowl Stovetop Lentil Casserole (page 80)

1 small plate vegetable salad

2 shakes low-fat salad dressing

1 small dinner roll

1 teaspoon butter

Snack

1 frozen fruit juice bar

There's an old saying: Prior planning prevents poor performance. That truism applies to food shopping, too. If you have a set list before you go to the grocery store, you'll be much less likely to buy high-calorie, low-nutrition foods. And not only will you and your family's health benefit, so will your budget.

Breakfast   time:

What I ate _____

_____

What I was doing while I ate

_____

Hunger level _____

Lunch   time:

What I ate _____

_____

What I was doing while I ate

_____

Hunger level _____

Dinner   time:

What I ate _____

_____

What I was doing while I ate

_____

Hunger level _____

Snack   time:

What I ate _____

_____

What I was doing while I ate

_____

Hunger level _____

Water

Remember to drink 8 glasses of water

I feel ___ about how I ate today:

☐ satisfied

☐ proud

☐ disappointed

☐ other _____

My goals for tomorrow:

_____

_____

_____

172

Walk the **Weight** Away!

Workout Journal

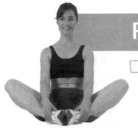

Pre-Walk Warm-Up

☐ **Spend 5 to 10 minutes slowly swinging your arms to prepare for your workout.**

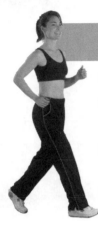

Walking Workout

Choose one.

☐ **Distance: 2 miles**
(15-minute-per-mile pace)

☐ **Time: 30 min.**
(15-minute-per-mile pace)

☐ **Steps: 4000 steps**

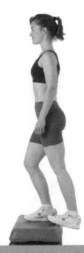

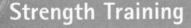

Strength Training

(1 set of 10 to 15 repetitions)

☐ **Shoulders Up,** page 118
☐ **Arm Power I,** page 119
☐ **Front Fly,** page 125
☐ **Back Fly,** page 122
☐ **Thigh Shaper,** page 126
☐ **Best Butt,** page 127
☐ **Six Pack,** page 132
☐ **Basic Crunch,** page 133

Post-Walk Stretches

☐ **Neck Stretch,** page 107
☐ **Shoulder Stretch,** page 108
☐ **Chest & Biceps Stretch,** page 110
☐ **Triceps Stretch,** page 109
☐ **Hamstring Stretch,** page 114
☐ **Quad Stretch,** page 113
☐ **Calf Stretch,** page 115

I feel __ about my workout today:

☐ satisfied
☐ proud
☐ disappointed
☐ other _____

My goals for tomorrow:

_____

_____

_____

Quote of the Day
Plan for success.
—Anonymous

Trainer's Tip
Keep your workout fun and interesting by varying the route of your walk.

173

Part 2
Walk the Weight Away!,
Day by Day

Nutrition Guide

Suggested Menu

Breakfast

1 small container non-fat yogurt mixed with 2 heaping tablespoons Grapenuts cereal

1 cup grapefruit juice

Lunch

• 1 Chicken Salad Sandwich Italiano (page 55)

1 cup grapes

1 handful raw baby carrots

Dinner

• 1 ½ cups Thai Pasta Salad (page 91)

1 small plate mixed berries

1 small dinner roll

1 teaspoon butter

Snack

1 handful dried fruit

When you're trying to improve your eating habits, don't expect to change everything you eat overnight. Set your sights on one habit at a time. For instance, you might concentrate on eating more fruit or even simply eating more slowly.

Breakfast   time:

What I ate _____

_____

What I was doing while I ate

_____

Hunger level _____

Lunch   time:

What I ate _____

_____

What I was doing while I ate

_____

Hunger level _____

Dinner   time:

What I ate _____

_____

What I was doing while I ate

_____

Hunger level _____

Snack   time:

What I ate _____

_____

What I was doing while I ate

_____

Hunger level _____

Water 🥛🥛🥛🥛🥛🥛🥛🥛🥛

Remember to drink 8 glasses of water

I feel __ about how I ate today:

☐ satisfied

☐ proud

☐ disappointed

☐ other _____

My goals for tomorrow:

_____

_____

_____

174

Walk
the
Weight
Away!

Workout Journal

Daily Stretches

- [ ] Head & Neck Stretch, page 107
- [ ] Shoulder Stretch, page 108
- [ ] Triceps Stretch, page 109
- [ ] Chest & Biceps Stretch, page 110
- [ ] Upper Back Stretch, page 111
- [ ] The Egg, page 112
- [ ] Quadriceps Stretch, page 113
- [ ] Hamstring Stretch, page 114
- [ ] Calf Stretch, page 115
- [ ] Butterfly Stretch, page 116

Chase the Chafe

If you experience a bit of inner thigh chafing as you walk, you're not alone. Avoiding cotton shorts or pants can help alleviate the problem. Another solution is to use one of the products on the market designed especially for the problem—Body Glide and petroleum jelly are popular choices.

Collect Your Favorites

Once you've been walking a couple of weeks, you'll probably start to "collect" favorite routes. Some walkers like to organize information about those routes in a notebook (or computer file). Some items you may want to track are the mileage of the route, special features ("plenty of water fountains" or "lots of puddles after rain"). That way, when you're getting bored with your usual walking route, you can refer back to your notes for an alternative.

Dry Up

Of course, you shouldn't let a little rain keep you from taking your walk, but how do you deal with those wet walking shoes? Place them in a dry spot and stuff them with newspaper. Once the newspaper is wet, just replace it.

Quote of the Day

While we may not be able to control all that happens to us, we can control what happens inside us.
—Benjamin Franklin

175

Part 2
Walk the Weight Away!,
Day by Day

Nutrition Guide

Suggested Menu

Breakfast

- Cheesy Potato Omelette (page 48)

1 slice whole wheat toast with 1 teaspoon butter

¼ cantaloupe

Lunch

- 1 cup Chicken & Sundried Tomato Pasta Salad (page 64)

1 cup non-fat milk

1 orange

Dinner

- 1 bowl Spunky Vegetarian Chili (page 79)

4 saltines

1 small plate vegetable salad

2 shakes low–fat salad dressing

Snack

6 to 8 whole grain crackers

176

Walk the Weight Away!

Everyone knows that setting goals is important for success. But to be useful, your goals must be specific and realistic. A better goal than "never overeating again" would be "not to eat ice cream this week."

Breakfast   time:

What I ate _____

_____

What I was doing while I ate

_____

Hunger level _____

Lunch   time:

What I ate _____

_____

What I was doing while I ate

_____

Hunger level _____

Dinner   time:

What I ate _____

_____

What I was doing while I ate

_____

Hunger level _____

Snack   time:

What I ate _____

_____

What I was doing while I ate

_____

Hunger level _____

Water

Remember to drink 8 glasses of water

I feel ___ about how I ate today:

- ☐ satisfied
- ☐ proud
- ☐ disappointed
- ☐ other _____

My goals for tomorrow:

_____

_____

_____

Workout Journal

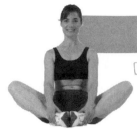

Pre-Walk Warm-Up

☐ **Spend 5 to 10 minutes slowly swinging your arms to prepare for your workout.**

Walking Workout

Choose one.

☐ **Distance: 2 miles**
(15-minute-per-mile pace)

☐ **Time: 30 min.**
(15-minute-per-mile pace)

☐ **Steps: 4000 steps**

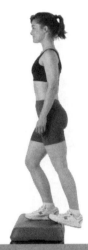

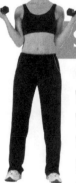

Strength Training

(1 set of 10 to 15 repetitions)
☐ **Arm Power II,** page 120
☐ **Tri Blaster,** page 121
☐ **Karate Kick,** page 128
☐ **Plié Press,** page 129
☐ **Hot Calves,** page 130
☐ **Strong Center,** page 131
☐ **Crunch Combo,** page 134

Post-Walk Stretches

☐ **Neck Stretch,** page 107
☐ **Chest & Biceps Stretch,**
page 110
☐ **Triceps Stretch,** page 109
☐ **Hamstring Stretch,** page 114
☐ **Quad Stretch,** page 113
☐ **Calf Stretch,** page 115

I feel __ about my workout today:
☐ satisfied
☐ proud
☐ disappointed
☐ other _____

My goals for tomorrow:

_____

_____

_____

Quote of the Day
Pick battles big enough to matter, small enough to win.
—Jonathan Kozol

Trainer's Tip
To add some extra cardio benefit to your workout walk intervals of "sprints"; that is, increase your walking speed for a few blocks and then return to your regular pace.

177

Part 2
Walk the Weight Away!,
Day by Day

Nutrition Guide

Suggested Menu

Breakfast

1 bowl high-fiber cereal

1 cup non-fat milk

1 handful nuts

Lunch

• 1 cup Spunky
Vegetarian Chili (page 79)

2 saltines

2 raw apricots

Dinner

• ½ plate Pot Roast
and Vegetables (page 76)

• ½ plate Spinach Salad
(page 90)

1 individual container
applesauce

Snack

1 banana

A road trip to Grandma's doesn't have to include a stop at a fast food restaurant. Instead, make sandwiches at home using healthful ingredients and pack snacks such as low-fat yogurt and carrot sticks. If the kids just won't sit still until they've had ice cream, stop for low-fat frozen yogurt instead.

Breakfast   time:

What I ate _____

_____

What I was doing while I ate

_____

Hunger level _____

Lunch   time:

What I ate _____

_____

What I was doing while I ate

_____

Hunger level _____

Dinner   time:

What I ate _____

_____

What I was doing while I ate

_____

Hunger level _____

Snack   time:

What I ate _____

_____

What I was doing while I ate

_____

Hunger level _____

Water

Remember to drink 8 glasses of water

I feel __ about how I ate today:

☐ satisfied

☐ proud

☐ disappointed

☐ other _____

My goals for tomorrow:

_____

_____

_____

178

Walk
the
Weight
Away!

Workout Journal

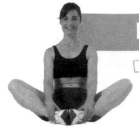

Pre-Walk Warm-Up

☐ **Spend 5 to 10 minutes slowly swinging your arms to prepare for your workout.**

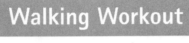

Walking Workout

Choose one.

☐ **Distance: 2 miles**
(15-minute-per-mile pace)

☐ **Time: 30 min.**
(15-minute-per-mile pace)

☐ **Steps: 4000 steps**

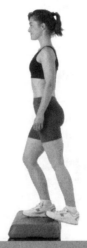

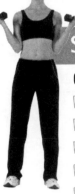

Strength Training

(1 set of 10 to 15 repetitions)
☐ **Shoulders Up,** page 118
☐ **Arm Power I,** page 119
☐ **Front Fly,** page 125
☐ **Back Fly,** page 122
☐ **Thigh Shaper,** page 126
☐ **Best Butt,** page 127
☐ **Six Pack,** page 132
☐ **Basic Crunch,** page 133

Post-Walk Stretches

☐ **Neck Stretch,** page 107
☐ **Shoulder Stretch,** page 108
☐ **Chest & Biceps Stretch,** page 110
☐ **Upper Back Stretch,** page 111
☐ **Hamstring Stretch,** page 114
☐ **Quad Stretch,** page 113
☐ **Calf Stretch,** page 115

I feel __ about my workout today:
☐ satisfied
☐ proud
☐ disappointed
☐ other _____

My goals for tomorrow:
_____
_____
_____

Quote of the Day
We aim above the mark to hit the mark.
—Ralph Waldo Emerson

Trainer's Tip
Walking during the morning or late afternoon or early evening hours are best to avoid exposure to the sun's UV rays.

179

Part 2
Walk the Weight Away!,
Day by Day

Nutrition Guide

Suggested Menu

Breakfast

2 packets instant oatmeal

1 small box raisins

1 cup non-fat milk

Lunch

- 1 Better-than-Pizza Potato (page 82)

1 plum

Dinner

- 1 Kielbasa Kebab (page 71)

1 small baked sweet potato sprayed with non-fat butter spray and sprinkled with cinnamon

1 small salad

2 shakes non-fat salad dressing

Snack

3 crackers with 1 teaspoon peanut butter

Do you like to come home from work and open a cold beer? Be careful—alcohol is packed with empty calories. If you don't want to give up your evening brew, switch to lite beer instead.

Breakfast   time:

What I ate _____

_____

What I was doing while I ate

_____

Hunger level _____

Lunch   time:

What I ate _____

_____

What I was doing while I ate

_____

Hunger level _____

Dinner   time:

What I ate _____

_____

What I was doing while I ate

_____

Hunger level _____

Snack   time:

What I ate _____

_____

What I was doing while I ate

_____

Hunger level _____

Water

Remember to drink 8 glasses of water

I feel __ about how I ate today:

☐ satisfied

☐ proud

☐ disappointed

☐ other _____

My goals for tomorrow:

_____

_____

_____

180

Walk the **Weight Away!**

Workout Journal

Daily Stretches

- ☐ Head & Neck Stretch, page 107
- ☐ Shoulder Stretch, page 108
- ☐ Triceps Stretch, page 109
- ☐ Chest & Biceps Stretch, page 110
- ☐ Upper Back Stretch, page 111

- ☐ The Egg, page 112
- ☐ Quadriceps Stretch, page 113
- ☐ Hamstring Stretch, page 114
- ☐ Calf Stretch, page 115
- ☐ Butterfly Stretch, page 116

Dress the Part

Let's face it: There are going to be days when you just don't feel like walking. When that happens, tell yourself that you'll just get dressed for your walk, but that you don't actually have to go. By the time you're dressed, we'll bet you head out for your walk after all.

Walk Smart on Treadmills

Walking on a treadmill can be intimidating if you've never tried it. But walking on one is easy and safe if you know what you're doing. One important tip to remember: Keep your body facing forward and don't look around as you walk. Twisting and turning your body makes it easy to lose your balance and fall.

Protect Your Skin

Using sunscreen is always a good idea when you walk. Don't forget to apply some to your ears and the back of your neck.

Quote of the Day

Striving for success without hard work is like trying to harvest where you haven't planted.
—David Bly

181

Part 2
Walk the Weight Away!,
Day by Day

Nutrition Guide

Suggested Menu

Breakfast

2 slices whole-grain toast

2 teaspoons jam

½ pint scrambled egg substitute, scrambled

½ grapefruit

Lunch

1 non-fat yogurt

1 cup strawberries

Dinner

• 1 piece Buttery Almond Fish (page 62)

¼ plate brown rice

½ plate broccoli

1 cup non-fat milk

Snack

2 handfuls raw vegetables with 2 shakes reduced fat salad dressing.

If you like to nibble throughout the day, break your meals into smaller portions and spread them out over the course of the day. It keeps your engine fueled and your taste buds satisfied.

Breakfast   time:

What I ate _____

_____

What I was doing while I ate

_____

Hunger level _____

Lunch   time:

What I ate _____

_____

What I was doing while I ate

_____

Hunger level _____

Dinner   time:

What I ate _____

_____

What I was doing while I ate

_____

Hunger level _____

Snack   time:

What I ate _____

_____

What I was doing while I ate

_____

Hunger level _____

Water

Remember to drink 8 glasses of water

I feel ___ about how I ate today:

☐ satisfied

☐ proud

☐ disappointed

☐ other _____

My goals for tomorrow:

_____

_____

_____

182

Walk
the
Weight
Away!

Workout Journal

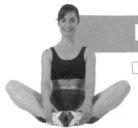

Pre-Walk Warm-Up

☐ **Spend 5 to 10 minutes slowly swinging your arms to prepare for your workout.**

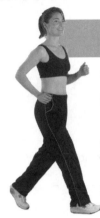

Walking Workout

Choose one.

☐ **Distance: 2.5 miles**
(15-minute-per-mile pace)

☐ **Time: 38 min.**
(15-minute-per-mile pace)

☐ **Steps: 5000 steps**

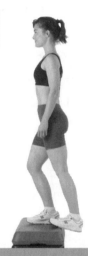

Strength Training

(1 set of 10 to 15 repetitions)

☐ **Arm Power II,** page 120
☐ **Tri Blaster,** page 121
☐ **Karate Kick,** page 128
☐ **Plié Press,** page 129
☐ **Hot Calves,** page 130
☐ **Strong Center,** page 131
☐ **Crunch Combo,** page 134

Post-Walk Stretches

☐ **Neck Stretch,** page 107
☐ **Chest & Biceps Stretch,** page 110
☐ **Triceps Stretch,** page 109
☐ **Hamstring Stretch,** page 114
☐ **Quad Stretch,** page 113
☐ **Calf Stretch,** page 115

I feel __ about my workout today:

☐ satisfied
☐ proud
☐ disappointed
☐ other _____

My goals for tomorrow:

_____
_____
_____

Quote of the Day

You are never given a wish without also being given the power to make it come true. You may have to work for it, however.
—Richard Bach

Trainer's Tip

As you stretch, breathe deeply and, after a few seconds of holding try to take the stretch a little deeper.

183

Part 2
Walk the Weight Away!,
Day by Day

Nutrition Guide

Suggested Menu

Breakfast

½ large bagel

2 heaping teaspoons peanut butter

1 small box raisins

1 cup non-fat milk

Lunch

• 1 Brunch Wrap (page 47)

1 handful baby carrots

1 cup non-fat milk

Dinner

• 1 bowl Cheese Ravioli Soup (page 63)

1 small vegetable salad

2 shakes low-fat salad dressing

1 small dinner roll

1 teaspoon butter

Snack

2 handfuls of popcorn or 2 rice cakes

184

Walk the Weight Away!

The importance of eating fruits and vegetables can't be overstated. Research shows that by eating at least five servings of the healthiest vegetables (for example, those that are dark green) and fruits each day, you can protect yourself from a variety of diseases, including several cancers. In addition to being rich in vitamins and other healthful substances, vegetables and fruits contain antioxidants, which work to undo damage caused to cells by free radicals.

Breakfast   time:

What I ate _____

_____

What I was doing while I ate

_____

Hunger level _____

Lunch   time:

What I ate _____

_____

What I was doing while I ate

_____

Hunger level _____

Dinner   time:

What I ate _____

_____

What I was doing while I ate

_____

Hunger level _____

Snack   time:

What I ate _____

_____

What I was doing while I ate

_____

Hunger level _____

Water

Remember to drink 8 glasses of water

I feel ___ about how I ate today:

☐ satisfied

☐ proud

☐ disappointed

☐ other _____

My goals for tomorrow:

_____

_____

_____

Workout Journal

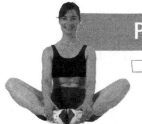

Pre-Walk Warm-Up

- ☐ Spend 5 to 10 minutes slowly swinging your arms to prepare for your workout.

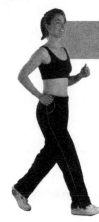

Walking Workout

Choose one.

- ☐ **Distance: 2.5 miles**
  (15-minute-per-mile pace)
- ☐ **Time: 38 min.**
  (15-minute-per-mile pace)
- ☐ **Steps: 5000 steps**

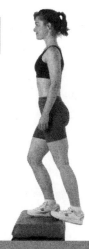

Strength Training

(1 set of 10 to 15 repetitions)

- ☐ **Shoulders Up,** page 118
- ☐ **Arm Power I,** page 119
- ☐ **Front Fly,** page 125
- ☐ **Modified Push-Up,** page 123
- ☐ **Back Fly,** page 122
- ☐ **Thigh Shaper,** page 126
- ☐ **Best Butt,** page 127
- ☐ **Six Pack,** page 132
- ☐ **Basic Crunch,** page 133

Post-Walk Stretches

- ☐ **Neck Stretch,** page 107
- ☐ **Shoulder Stretch,** page 108
- ☐ **Chest & Biceps Stretch,** page 110
- ☐ **Upper Back Stretch,** page 111
- ☐ **Hamstring Stretch,** page 114
- ☐ **Quad Stretch,** page 113
- ☐ **Calf Stretch,** page 115

I feel ___ about my workout today:

- ☐ satisfied
- ☐ proud
- ☐ disappointed
- ☐ other _____

My goals for tomorrow:

_____

_____

_____

Quote of the Day

Human beings, by changing the inner attitudes of their minds, can change the outer aspects of their lives.
—William James

Trainer's Tip

If you miss a session don't despair. Just add an extra walking session next week.

185

Part 2
Walk the Weight Away!,
Day by Day

Phase 2: Commitment

Nutrition Guide

Suggested Menu

Breakfast

- 1 Graham Cracker Muffin (page 50)

  1 cup non-fat milk

  1 small banana

Lunch

- 1 small plate Waldorf Salad (page 92)

  4 saltines

Dinner

- 1 Updated Sloppy Joe Sandwich (page 58)

  ¼ plate cooked corn

  ½ plate vegetable salad

  2 shakes low-fat salad dressing

Snack

  1 bag light microwave popcorn

186

Walk the **Weight** Away!

You've probably heard someone say something like, "I was so bad yesterday," meaning that she overate. Try not to label yourself as "bad" when you fall short of one of your goals. Not only is it not helpful, but it's actually discouraging.

Breakfast   time:

What I ate _____

_____

What I was doing while I ate

_____

Hunger level _____

Lunch   time:

What I ate _____

_____

What I was doing while I ate

_____

Hunger level _____

Dinner   time:

What I ate _____

_____

What I was doing while I ate

_____

Hunger level _____

Snack   time:

What I ate _____

_____

What I was doing while I ate

_____

Hunger level _____

Water ⬚⬚⬚⬚⬚⬚⬚⬚⬚⬚

Remember to drink 8 glasses of water

I feel __ about how I ate today:

☐ satisfied

☐ proud

☐ disappointed

☐ other _____

My goals for tomorrow:

_____

_____

_____

Workout Journal

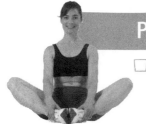

Pre-Walk Warm-Up

☐ **Spend 5 to 10 minutes slowly swinging your arms to prepare for your workout.**

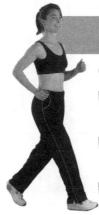

Walking Workout

Choose one.

☐ **Distance: 2.5 miles**
(15-minute-per-mile pace)

☐ **Time: 38 min.**
(15-minute-per-mile pace)

☐ **Steps: 5000 steps**

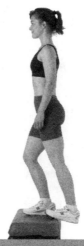

Strength Training

(1 set of 10 to 15 repetitions)

☐ **Arm Power II,** page 120
☐ **Tri Blaster,** page 121
☐ **Karate Kick,** page 128
☐ **Plié Press,** page 129
☐ **Hot Calves,** page 130
☐ **Strong Center,** page 131
☐ **Crunch Combo,** page 134

Post-Walk Stretches

☐ **Neck Stretch,** page 107
☐ **Chest & Biceps Stretch,** page 110
☐ **Triceps Stretch,** page 109
☐ **Upper Back Stretch,** page 111
☐ **Hamstring Stretch,** page 114
☐ **Quad Stretch,** page 113
☐ **Calf Stretch,** page 115

I feel ___ about my workout today:
☐ satisfied
☐ proud
☐ disappointed
☐ other _____

My goals for tomorrow:
_____
_____
_____

Quote of the Day
Our greatest glory is not in never failing, but in rising every time we fail.
—Confucius

Trainer's Tip
To increase the likelihood of sticking to your routine, make your walking time and place as convenient as possible for you.

187

Part 2
Walk the Weight Away!, Day by Day

Nutrition Guide

Suggested Menu

Breakfast

1 bowl high-fiber cereal

1 cup non-fat milk

1 handful nuts

Lunch

2 slices rye bread

3 slices deli turkey breast

1 tablespoon low-fat mayonnaise

lettuce and tomato

1 handful baked chips

1 handful blueberries

Dinner

- 1 piece Chicken Del Jardin (page 66)

¼ plate couscous

- ¼ plate Roasted Carrots with Lime (page 88)

Snack

1 large handful grapes

It's never a good idea to eat a big meal just before working out. If you feel that you need a snack, have a banana. Bananas are filling, easy to digest, and give you quick energy.

Breakfast   time:

What I ate _____

_____

What I was doing while I ate

_____

Hunger level _____

Lunch   time:

What I ate _____

_____

What I was doing while I ate

_____

Hunger level _____

Dinner   time:

What I ate _____

_____

What I was doing while I ate

_____

Hunger level _____

Snack   time:

What I ate _____

_____

What I was doing while I ate

_____

Hunger level _____

Water 🥤🥤🥤🥤🥤🥤🥤🥤

Remember to drink 8 glasses of water

I feel ___ about how I ate today:

☐ satisfied

☐ proud

☐ disappointed

☐ other _____

My goals for tomorrow:

_____

_____

_____

188

Walk the **Weight Away!**

Workout Journal

Daily Stretches

- ☐ Head & Neck Stretch, page 107
- ☐ Shoulder Stretch, page 108
- ☐ Triceps Stretch, page 109
- ☐ Chest & Biceps Stretch, page 110
- ☐ Upper Back Stretch, page 111
- ☐ The Egg, page 112
- ☐ Quadriceps Stretch, page 113
- ☐ Hamstring Stretch, page 114
- ☐ Calf Stretch, page 115
- ☐ Butterfly Stretch, page 116

Love Your Feet

If you've been sedentary for a long time, you will definitely want to give your feet a little extra care when you start a walking program. Pay special attention to your toenails; keep them trimmed straight, but not too short. And if your feet perspire a lot, keep foot powder handy.

Make an Appointment with Yourself

Consistency is key especially when you're just starting an exercise program. Block out time in your day to exercise just as you would for any other important appointment and you'll be more likely to stick with it.

Don't Skimp on Sleep

Sleep is as important to your fitness program as exercise. It gives you the energy you need to walk with vigor, and that allows you to burn more calories.

Quote of the Day

The first and most important step toward success is the feeling that we can succeed.
—Nelson Boswell

189

Part 2
Walk the Weight Away!,
Day by Day

Nutrition Guide

Suggested Menu

Breakfast

2 slices whole-grain toast

2 teaspoons jam

½ pint scrambled egg substitute, scrambled

½ grapefruit

Lunch

2 slices whole grain bread

2 slices deli roast beef

1 tablespoon light mayonnaise

lettuce and tomato

1 pear

Dinner

• ½ plate Spaghetti Squash Pomodoro (page 78)

• ½ plate Spinach Salad (page 90)

1 small dinner roll

1 teaspoon butter

Snack

1 cup fruit juice

190

Walk the Weight Away!

To increase your supply of healthful, low-fat recipes, organize a recipe swap with your friends and family members. Of course, you don't necessarily have to give up all your favorite recipes. Computer programs that perform nutritional analysis on recipes are widely available and inexpensive.

Breakfast   time:

What I ate _____

_____

What I was doing while I ate

_____

Hunger level _____

Lunch   time:

What I ate _____

_____

What I was doing while I ate

_____

Hunger level _____

Dinner   time:

What I ate _____

_____

What I was doing while I ate

_____

Hunger level _____

Snack   time:

What I ate _____

_____

What I was doing while I ate

_____

Hunger level _____

Water

Remember to drink 8 glasses of water

I feel ___ about how I ate today:

☐ satisfied

☐ proud

☐ disappointed

☐ other _____

My goals for tomorrow:

_____

_____

_____

Workout Journal

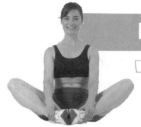

Pre-Walk Warm-Up

☐ Spend 5 to 10 minutes slowly swinging your arms to prepare for your workout.

Walking Workout

Choose one.

☐ **Distance: 2.5 miles**
(15-minute-per-mile pace)

☐ **Time: 38 min.**
(15-minute-per-mile pace)

☐ **Steps: 5000 steps**

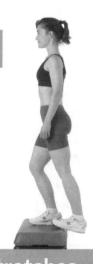

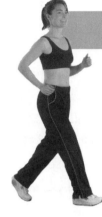

Strength Training

(1 set of 10 to 15 repetitions)

☐ **Shoulders Up,** page 118
☐ **Arm Power I,** page 119
☐ **Front Fly,** page 125
☐ **Modified Push-Up,** page 123
☐ **Back Fly,** page 122
☐ **Thigh Shaper,** page 126
☐ **Best Butt,** page 127
☐ **Six Pack,** page 132
☐ **Basic Crunch,** page 133

Post-Walk Stretches

☐ **Neck Stretch,** page 107
☐ **Chest & Biceps Stretch,**
page 110
☐ **Triceps Stretch,** page 109
☐ **Upper Back Stretch,** page 111
☐ **Hamstring Stretch,** page 114
☐ **Quad Stretch,** page 113
☐ **Calf Stretch,** page 115

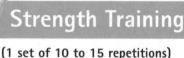

I feel __ about my workout today:

☐ satisfied
☐ proud
☐ disappointed
☐ other _____

My goals for tomorrow:

_____

_____

_____

Quote of the Day
Victory belongs to the most persevering.
—Napoleon Bonaparte

Trainer's Tip
Reward yourself after your workouts with a nice hot bath or soothing massage.

191

Part 2
*Walk the
Weight Away!,*
Day by Day

Nutrition Guide

Suggested Menu

Breakfast

1 small container non-fat yogurt mixed with 2 heaping tablespoons Grapenuts cereal

1 cup grapefruit juice

Lunch

1 small bagel with 2 slices lean ham, 1 slice low-fat cheese, and Dijon mustard

1 handful cherry tomatoes

1 peach

Dinner

- 1 piece Chicken Cacciatore (page 65)

¼ plate cooked bowtie pasta with sauce

1 small salad

2 shakes low-fat salad dressing

Snack

1 handful baked tortilla chips with salsa

192

Walk the Weight Away!

People tend to be more successful in their endeavors to lose weight and eat healthfully if they have community support. One way to find that support is to join a an online weight loss group where you can interact with other people who are trying to lose weight and eat more healthfully. To find such groups, search online using the keywords: "weight loss support."

Breakfast   time:

What I ate _____

_____

What I was doing while I ate

_____

Hunger level _____

Lunch   time:

What I ate _____

_____

What I was doing while I ate

_____

Hunger level _____

Dinner   time:

What I ate _____

_____

What I was doing while I ate

_____

Hunger level _____

Snack   time:

What I ate _____

_____

What I was doing while I ate

_____

Hunger level _____

Water

Remember to drink 8 glasses of water

I feel ___ about how I ate today:

- ☐ satisfied
- ☐ proud
- ☐ disappointed
- ☐ other _____

My goals for tomorrow:

_____

_____

_____

Workout Journal

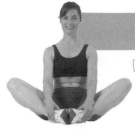

Pre-Walk Warm-Up

☐ **Spend 5 to 10 minutes slowly swinging your arms to prepare for your workout.**

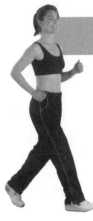

Walking Workout

Choose one.

☐ **Distance: 2.5 miles**
(15-minute-per-mile pace)

☐ **Time: 38 min.**
(15-minute-per-mile pace)

☐ **Steps: 5000 steps**

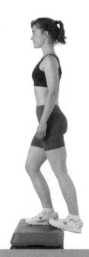

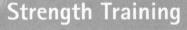

Strength Training

(1 set of 10 to 15 repetitions)

☐ **Arm Power II**, page 120
☐ **Tri Blaster**, page 121
☐ **Karate Kick**, page 128
☐ **Plié Press**, page 129
☐ **Hot Calves**, page 130
☐ **Strong Center**, page 131
☐ **Crunch Combo**, page 134

Post-Walk Stretches

☐ **Neck Stretch**, page 107
☐ **Chest & Biceps Stretch**, page 110
☐ **Triceps Stretch**, page 109
☐ **Upper Back Stretch**, page 111
☐ **Hamstring Stretch**, page 114
☐ **Quad Stretch**, page 113
☐ **Calf Stretch**, page 115

I feel __ about my workout today:

☐ satisfied
☐ proud
☐ disappointed
☐ other _____

My goals for tomorrow:

_____

_____

_____

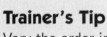

Quote of the Day

Do not wait; the time will never be "just right." Start where you stand, and work with whatever tools you may have at your command, and better tools will be found as you go along.
—Napoleon Hill

Trainer's Tip

Vary the order in which you perform your strength training exercises to "surprise" your muscles.

193

Nutrition Guide

Suggested Menu

Breakfast

- Strawberry Orange Muffin (page 52)

  1 banana

  1 cup non-fat milk

Lunch

- Updated Sloppy Joe Sandwich (page 58)

  1 orange

Dinner

- ¼ plate Teriyaki Steak Fingers (page 81)
- ¼ plate Smashed Potatoes (page 89)

  1 small vegetable salad

  2 shakes low-fat salad dressing

Snack

1 cup fresh berries

Are you a mindless nibbler, someone who reaches for snack food during the day just out of habit? Keep a bag of baby carrots on your desk at work or by your side at home. That way, you can accommodate your habit without putting on pounds.

Breakfast   time:

What I ate _____

_____

What I was doing while I ate

_____

Hunger level _____

Lunch   time:

What I ate _____

_____

What I was doing while I ate

_____

Hunger level _____

Dinner   time:

What I ate _____

_____

What I was doing while I ate

_____

Hunger level _____

Snack   time:

What I ate _____

_____

What I was doing while I ate

_____

Hunger level _____

Water

Remember to drink 8 glasses of water

I feel ___ about how I ate today:

- ☐ satisfied
- ☐ proud
- ☐ disappointed
- ☐ other _____

My goals for tomorrow:

_____

_____

_____

194

Walk the **Weight** Away!

Workout Journal

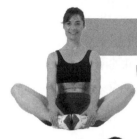

Pre-Walk Warm-Up

☐ **Spend 5 to 10 minutes slowly swinging your arms to prepare for your workout.**

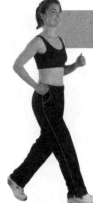

Walking Workout

Choose one.

☐ **Distance: 3 miles**
(15-minute-per-mile pace)

☐ **Time: 45 min.**
(15-minute-per-mile pace)

☐ **Steps: 6000 steps**

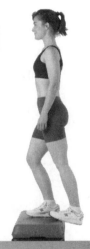

Strength Training

(1 set of 10 to 15 repetitions)

☐ **Shoulders Up,** page 118
☐ **Arm Power I,** page 119
☐ **Front Fly,** page 125
☐ **Modified Push-Up,** page 123
☐ **Back Fly,** page 122
☐ **Thigh Shaper,** page 126
☐ **Best Butt,** page 127
☐ **Six Pack,** page 132
☐ **Basic Crunch,** page 133

Post-Walk Stretches

☐ **Neck Stretch,** page 107
☐ **Chest & Biceps Stretch,** page 110
☐ **Triceps Stretch,** page 109
☐ **Upper Back Stretch,** page 111
☐ **Hamstring Stretch,** page 114
☐ **Quad Stretch,** page 113
☐ **Calf Stretch,** page 115

I feel ___ about my workout today:
☐ satisfied
☐ proud
☐ disappointed
☐ other _____

My goals for tomorrow:
_____
_____
_____

Quote of the Day
A happy person is not a person in a certain set of circumstances, but rather a person with a certain set of attitudes.
—Hugh Downs

Trainer's Tip
Never walk so fast that you feel you are out of breath or can't carry on a conversation. Let your heart rate be your guide.

195

Part 2
Walk the Weight Away!,
Day by Day

Nutrition Guide

Suggested Menu

Breakfast

- 1 Blueberry Muffin
  (page 46)
  1 small banana
  1 cup non-fat milk

Lunch

- 1 ½ cups Thai Pasta Salad
  (page 91)
  1 pear

Dinner

- 1 bowl Pasta Primavera
  (page 72)
  1 small vegetable salad
  2 shakes low-fat
  salad dressing
  1 slice Italian bread

Snack

2 large graham crackers

Don't underestimate the power of positive thinking. It may sound like a cliché, but it's true. Changing old habits is hard work, and keeping a positive mental attitude is important and helpful. Give yourself a pep talk now and then—even simple phrases like, "hang in there," and "You can do it," are effective.

Breakfast   time:

What I ate _____

_____

What I was doing while I ate

_____

Hunger level _____

Lunch   time:

What I ate _____

_____

What I was doing while I ate

_____

Hunger level _____

Dinner   time:

What I ate _____

_____

What I was doing while I ate

_____

Hunger level _____

Snack   time:

What I ate _____

_____

What I was doing while I ate

_____

Hunger level _____

Water

Remember to drink 8 glasses of water

I feel __ about how I ate today:

- ☐ satisfied
- ☐ proud
- ☐ disappointed
- ☐ other _____

My goals for tomorrow:

_____

_____

_____

196

Walk
the
Weight
Away!

Workout Journal

Daily Stretches

- [ ] Head & Neck Stretch, page 107
- [ ] Shoulder Stretch, page 108
- [ ] Triceps Stretch, page 109
- [ ] Chest & Biceps Stretch, page 110
- [ ] Upper Back Stretch, page 111

- [ ] The Egg, page 112
- [ ] Quadriceps Stretch, page 113
- [ ] Hamstring Stretch, page 114
- [ ] Calf Stretch, page 115
- [ ] Butterfly Stretch, page 116

Visit a Walking City!

According to the American Podiatric Medical Association (APMA), the ten top-rated cities for walking are: New York, San Francisco, Boston, Philadelphia, Seattle, Denver, Washington DC, Chicago, Portland, Ore., and Cleveland. The APMA says that these cities have many parks and the highest percentage of people who walk to work.

Hit the Trails

Sure, you can walk around the neighborhood or in a local park, but if you live near hiking trails, there are dozens of other options open to you. Hiking doesn't have to be strenuous; some trails are simply easy walks through forests. To find parks in your state, search online using your state's name and the word *parks*, for example: "Delaware State Parks".

Shorten Your Stride, Increase Your Speed

At this point you've been on the *Walk the Weight Away!* walking program for three weeks. Maybe you're looking to increase your pace. If so, do that by shortening your stride and quickening your steps—not by increasing your stride length, which can lead to injury.

Quote of the Day

It is difficult to say what is impossible, for the dream of yesterday is the hope of today and the reality of tomorrow.
—Robert H. Goddard

197

Part 2
Walk the Weight Away!,
Day by Day

Nutrition Guide

If your all-time favorite food is chocolate ice cream, it's foolish (and unrealistic) to think you can give it up forever. Making a food forbidden only makes it more tempting. Instead, plan to splurge on your favorite food once in a while. When you know you can have a favorite food, you'll be less likely to feel deprived, and when you don't feel deprived, changing the way you eat will be easier.

Suggested Menu

Breakfast

2 slices whole-grain toast

2 teaspoons jam

½ pint scrambled egg substitute, scrambled

½ grapefruit

Lunch

• 1 cup Chunky Beef & Vegetable Soup (page 67)

½ bagel

1 teaspoon butter

Dinner

• 1 bowl Stovetop Lentil Casserole (page 80)

1 small plate vegetable salad

2 shakes low-fat salad dressing

1 small dinner roll

1 teaspoon butter

Snack

1 slice string cheese with 3 crackers

Breakfast   time:

What I ate _____

_____

What I was doing while I ate

_____

Hunger level _____

Lunch   time:

What I ate _____

_____

What I was doing while I ate

_____

Hunger level _____

Dinner   time:

What I ate _____

_____

What I was doing while I ate

_____

Hunger level _____

Snack   time:

What I ate _____

_____

What I was doing while I ate

_____

Hunger level _____

Water

Remember to drink 8 glasses of water

I feel ___ about how I ate today:

☐ satisfied

☐ proud

☐ disappointed

☐ other _____

My goals for tomorrow:

_____

_____

_____

198

Walk the **Weight** Away!

Workout Journal

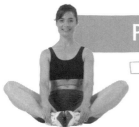

Pre-Walk Warm-Up

☐ **Spend 5 to 10 minutes slowly swinging your arms to prepare for your workout.**

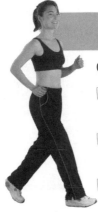

Walking Workout

Choose one.

☐ **Distance: 3 miles**
(15-minute-per-mile pace)

☐ **Time: 45 min.**
(15-minute-per-mile pace)

☐ **Steps: 6000 steps**

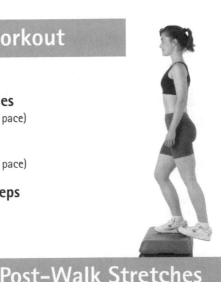

Strength Training

(2 set of 10 to 15 repetitions)
☐ **Arm Power II**, page 120
☐ **Tri Blaster**, page 121
☐ **Karate Kick**, page 128
☐ **Plié Press**, page 129
☐ **Hot Calves**, page 130
☐ **Strong Center**, page 131
☐ **Crunch Combo**, page 134

Post-Walk Stretches

☐ **Neck Stretch**, page 107
☐ **Chest & Biceps Stretch**, page 110
☐ **Triceps Stretch**, page 109
☐ **Upper Back Stretch**, page 111
☐ **Hamstring Stretch**, page 114
☐ **Quad Stretch**, page 113
☐ **Calf Stretch**, page 115

I feel ___ about my workout today:
☐ satisfied
☐ proud
☐ disappointed
☐ other _____

My goals for tomorrow:

_____

_____

_____

Quote of the Day
Edison failed 10,000 times before perfecting the incandescent electric light bulb. Don't worry if you fail once. —Napoleon Hill

Trainer's Tip
When weight training, be careful never to lift weights too quickly or you will both increase your risk for injury and involve momentum more than muscle. Try counting to two as you lift, and to four as you lower.

199

Part 2
***Walk the Weight Away!*,**
Day by Day

Nutrition Guide

Suggested Menu

Breakfast
- Greek Omelette (page 51)
  - ½ English muffin
  - 1 teaspoon jam
  - 1 cup berries

Lunch
- 1 plate Spinach Salad (page 90)
  - 1 handful grapes
  - ½ small whole grain bagel
  - 1 teaspoon butter

Dinner
- ¾ cup Barbecued Pork (page 61)
  - 1 whole grain hamburger bun
  - 1 cup vegetable salad
  - 1 small watermelon wedge

Snack
- 1 container non-fat yogurt

Eating salad is a wonderful way to get your vegetables, especially if you load it up with dark, green leafy vegetables. The trouble comes in when you also load it up with salad dressing. Some dressing have as much as 100 calories in a tablespoon—and how many of us use just one tablespoon of dressing?

One way to eliminate the calories on your next salad is to dress it only with a sprinkling of balsamic vinegar, a vinegar from Italy that adds loads of flavor—but almost no calories—to most any salad.

Breakfast   time:

What I ate _____

_____

What I was doing while I ate

_____

Hunger level _____

Lunch   time:

What I ate _____

_____

What I was doing while I ate

_____

Hunger level _____

Dinner   time:

What I ate _____

_____

What I was doing while I ate

_____

Hunger level _____

Snack   time:

What I ate _____

_____

What I was doing while I ate

_____

Hunger level _____

Water ⊍⊍⊍⊍⊍⊍⊍⊍
Remember to drink 8 glasses of water

I feel ___ about how I ate today:
- ☐ satisfied
- ☐ proud
- ☐ disappointed
- ☐ other _____

My goals for tomorrow:

_____

_____

_____

200

Walk
the
Weight
Away!

Workout Journal

Daily Stretches

☐ Head & Neck Stretch, page 107
☐ Shoulder Stretch, page 108
☐ Triceps Stretch, page 109
☐ Chest & Biceps Stretch, page 110
☐ Upper Back Stretch, page 111

☐ The Egg, page 112
☐ Quadriceps Stretch, page 113
☐ Hamstring Stretch, page 114
☐ Calf Stretch, page 115
☐ Butterfly Stretch, page 116

Relax Your Mind

Do you find yourself ruminating over the problems of the day during your walk? Instead, try to use the time to relax and focus on the scenery. Often, it's when your mind is relaxed that solutions to problems emerge.

Work Your Abs While You Walk

Improve your posture and tighten your tummy by pulling in your abs as you walk.

More Good News

According to the government, some weight-loss and conditioning studies have shown that walking is more effective than running and other more highly-touted activities. That's because there's virtually no risk of injury and it has the lowest dropout rate of any form of exercise.

Quote of the Day
What lies behind us and what lies before us are tiny matters compared to what lies within us.
—Ralph Waldo Emerson

201

Part 2
Walk the Weight Away!,
Day by Day

Nutrition Guide

Suggested Menu

Breakfast

- 2 slices French Toast (page 49)

  1 orange

  1 slice Canadian bacon

Lunch

- 1 Strawberry Orange Muffin (page 52)

  1 apple

  1 small container non-fat, no sugar added yogurt

Dinner

1 low-fat hotdog

1 hotdog roll

1 handful low-fat chips

¼ plate baked beans

Snack

½ baked potato with salsa

You probably keep certain staples, like bread and milk, on hand in your kitchen. Here are two more items to add to that list: bags of frozen mixed vegetables and cans or cartons of fat-free chicken broth. When you need a quick, healthy dinner, just combine some broth and vegetables and heat until the broth and vegetables are heated through.

Breakfast   time:

What I ate _____

_____

What I was doing while I ate

_____

Hunger level _____

Lunch   time:

What I ate _____

_____

What I was doing while I ate

_____

Hunger level _____

Dinner   time:

What I ate _____

_____

What I was doing while I ate

_____

Hunger level _____

Snack   time:

What I ate _____

_____

What I was doing while I ate

_____

Hunger level _____

Water

Remember to drink 8 glasses of water

I feel ___ about how I ate today:

- ☐ satisfied
- ☐ proud
- ☐ disappointed
- ☐ other _____

My goals for tomorrow:

_____

_____

_____

202

Walk the Weight Away!

Workout Journal

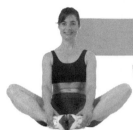

Pre-Walk Warm-Up

☐ **Spend 5 to 10 minutes slowly swinging your arms to prepare for your workout.**

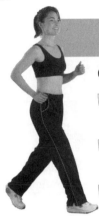

Walking Workout

Choose one.

☐ **Distance: 3 miles**
(15-minute-per-mile pace)

☐ **Time: 45 min.**
(15-minute-per-mile pace)

☐ **Steps: 6000 steps**

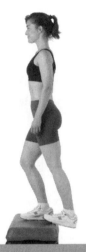

Strength Training

(2 set of 10 to 15 repetitions)
☐ **Shoulders Up,** page 118
☐ **Arm Power I,** page 119
☐ **Front Fly,** page 125
☐ **Modified Push-Up,** page 123
☐ **Back Fly,** page 122
☐ **Thigh Shaper,** page 126
☐ **Best Butt,** page 127
☐ **Six Pack,** page 132
☐ **Basic Crunch,** page 133

Post-Walk Stretches

☐ **Neck Stretch,** page 107
☐ **Chest & Biceps Stretch,** page 110
☐ **Triceps Stretch,** page 109
☐ **Upper Back Stretch,** page 111
☐ **Hamstring Stretch,** page 114
☐ **Quad Stretch,** page 113
☐ **Calf Stretch,** page 115

I feel ___ about my workout today:
☐ satisfied
☐ proud
☐ disappointed
☐ other _____

My goals for tomorrow:

_____

_____

_____

Quote of the Day
What we hope ever to do with ease we may learn first to do with diligence.
—Samuel Johnson

Trainer's Tip
If you injure a muscle follow the RICE treatment immediately: Rest, Ice, Compress (with a bandage), and Elevate the injured muscle.

203

Part 2
Walk the Weight Away!,
Day by Day

Nutrition Guide

Suggested Menu

Breakfast

1 bowl high-fiber cereal
1 cup non-fat milk
1 handful nuts

Lunch

2 slices whole grain bread
2 slices lean deli ham
1 slice low-fat cheese
1 tablespoon Dijon mustard
1 handful baked chips
1 handful fresh cherries

Dinner

- **1 piece Grilled Marinated Salmon** (page 70)
  - ¼ plate Rice Pilaf (page 87)
  - ½ plate Spinach Salad (page 90)

Snack

1 cup fresh berries

One of the best kitchen tool investments you can make is an oil mister, a refillable canister that lets you spray cooking oil onto foods. The advantage of a mister is that you can spray a very light coating—no more than absolutely necessary—onto foods before grilling. That saves calories and adds flavor that you won't find in many cooking sprays. You can find misters in most department stores.

Breakfast   time:

What I ate _____

_____

What I was doing while I ate

_____

Hunger level _____

Lunch   time:

What I ate _____

_____

What I was doing while I ate

_____

Hunger level _____

Dinner   time:

What I ate _____

_____

What I was doing while I ate

_____

Hunger level _____

Snack   time:

What I ate _____

_____

What I was doing while I ate

_____

Hunger level _____

Water

Remember to drink 8 glasses of water

I feel __ about how I ate today:

- ☐ satisfied
- ☐ proud
- ☐ disappointed
- ☐ other _____

My goals for tomorrow:

_____

_____

_____

204

Walk the **Weight** **Away!**

Workout Journal

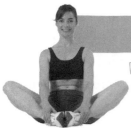

Pre-Walk Warm-Up

☐ **Spend 5 to 10 minutes slowly swinging your arms to prepare for your workout.**

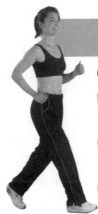

Walking Workout

Choose one.

☐ **Distance: 3 miles**
(15-minute-per-mile pace)

☐ **Time: 45 min.**
(15-minute-per-mile pace)

☐ **Steps: 6000 steps**

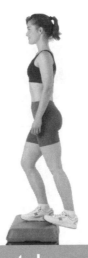

Strength Training

(2 set of 10 to 15 repetitions)
☐ **Arm Power II,** page 120
☐ **Tri Blaster,** page 121
☐ **Karate Kick,** page 128
☐ **Plié Press,** page 129
☐ **Hot Calves,** page 130
☐ **Strong Center,** page 131
☐ **Crunch Combo,** page 134

Post-Walk Stretches

☐ **Neck Stretch,** page 107
☐ **Chest & Biceps Stretch,** page 110
☐ **Triceps Stretch,** page 109
☐ **Upper Back Stretch,** page 111
☐ **Hamstring Stretch,** page 114
☐ **Quad Stretch,** page 113
☐ **Calf Stretch,** page 115

I feel __ about my workout today:
☐ satisfied
☐ proud
☐ disappointed
☐ other _____

My goals for tomorrow:

_____

_____

_____

Quote of the Day
Look well into thyself; there is a source of strength which will always spring up if thou wilt always look there.
—Marcus Aurelius Antoninus

Trainer's Tip
When walking around a track, do half your walk clockwise, the other counterclockwise. Continually walking in one direction can cause knee pain and injury.

205

Part 2
Walk the Weight Away!,
Day by Day

Nutrition Guide

Suggested Menu

Breakfast
- 3 Whole Wheat Pancakes with Strawberry Syrup (page 54, page 53)

  1 cup non-fat milk

Lunch
- 1 Heart-Healthy Egg Salad Sandwich (page 56)

  raw cucumber slices

  1 apple

Dinner
- 1 portion Southwestern Pork Tenderloin (page 77)

  1 ear corn

  ½ plate mixed vegetable salad

  1 tablespoon low-fat salad dressing

Snack
- 1 handful raw veggies dipped in Lemon Chickpea Hummus (page 57)

Going to a restaurant doesn't have to turn into an occasion to overeat. There are some strategies you can use to stay on track. First, skip the bread; not because carbohydrates are "bad," but because it adds extra calories before you even have your entrée. Second, ask that your food be boiled or sautéed in very little fat. Third, ask that any sauce be served on the side; that way, you can control how much you use. Finally, if you've gotta have dessert, stick to fresh fruit or sorbet.

Breakfast   time:

What I ate _____

_____

What I was doing while I ate

_____

Hunger level _____

Lunch   time:

What I ate _____

_____

What I was doing while I ate

_____

Hunger level _____

Dinner   time:

What I ate _____

_____

What I was doing while I ate

_____

Hunger level _____

Snack   time:

What I ate _____

_____

What I was doing while I ate

_____

Hunger level _____

Water

Remember to drink 8 glasses of water

I feel ___ about how I ate today:
- ☐ satisfied
- ☐ proud
- ☐ disappointed
- ☐ other _____

My goals for tomorrow:

_____

_____

_____

206

Walk the **Weight** Away!

Workout Journal

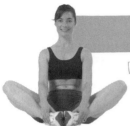

Pre-Walk Warm-Up

☐ **Spend 5 to 10 minutes slowly swinging your arms to prepare for your workout.**

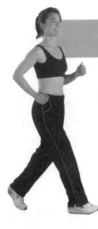

Walking Workout

Choose one.

☐ **Distance: 3 miles**
(15-minute-per-mile pace)

☐ **Time: 45 min.**
(15-minute-per-mile pace)

☐ **Steps: 6000 steps**

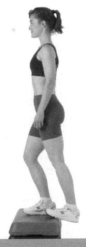

Strength Training

(2 set of 10 to 15 repetitions)

☐ **Shoulders Up,** page 118
☐ **Arm Power I,** page 119
☐ **Front Fly,** page 125
☐ **Modified Push-Up,** page 123
☐ **Back Fly,** page 122
☐ **Thigh Shaper,** page 126
☐ **Best Butt,** page 127
☐ **Six Pack,** page 132
☐ **Basic Crunch,** page 133

Post-Walk Stretches

☐ **Neck Stretch,** page 107
☐ **Chest & Biceps Stretch,** page 110
☐ **Triceps Stretch,** page 109
☐ **Upper Back Stretch,** page 111
☐ **Hamstring Stretch,** page 114
☐ **Quad Stretch,** page 113
☐ **Calf Stretch,** page 115

I feel __ about my workout today:

☐ satisfied
☐ proud
☐ disappointed
☐ other _____

My goals for tomorrow:

_____

_____

_____

Quote of the Day

In reality, serendipity accounts for one percent of the blessings we receive in life, work, and love. The other 99 percent is due to our efforts.
—Peter McWilliams

Trainer's Tip

When you weight train concentrate on squeezing the muscle you're working, and not the weight you're working with.

207

Part 2
Walk the Weight Away!,
Day by Day

Nutrition Guide

Suggested Menu

Breakfast

- Cheesy Potato Omelette (page 48)

1 slice whole wheat toast with 1 teaspoon butter

¼ cantaloupe

Lunch

- 1 cup Chicken & Sundried Tomato Pasta Salad (page 64)

1 cup non-fat milk

1 orange

Dinner

- 1 bowl Spunky Vegetarian Chili (page 79)

4 saltines

1 small plate vegetable salad

2 shakes low-fat salad dressing

Snack

1 frozen pancake with a squeeze of light syrup

208

Walk the Weight Away!

Wrap-style sandwiches are popular these days—we have even included a recipe for one in the *Walk the Weight Away!* collection. But use tortillas to make sandwiches only occasionally. They're higher in fat and calories than pita bread. There's no need to eliminate them from your diet; simply use them sparingly.

Breakfast   time:

What I ate _____

_____

What I was doing while I ate

_____

Hunger level _____

Lunch   time:

What I ate _____

_____

What I was doing while I ate

_____

Hunger level _____

Dinner   time:

What I ate _____

_____

What I was doing while I ate

_____

Hunger level _____

Snack   time:

What I ate _____

_____

What I was doing while I ate

_____

Hunger level _____

Water

Remember to drink 8 glasses of water

I feel ___ about how I ate today:

- ☐ satisfied
- ☐ proud
- ☐ disappointed
- ☐ other _____

My goals for tomorrow:

_____

_____

_____

Workout Journal

Daily Stretches

- ☐ Head & Neck Stretch, page 107
- ☐ Shoulder Stretch, page 108
- ☐ Triceps Stretch, page 109
- ☐ Chest & Biceps Stretch, page 110
- ☐ Upper Back Stretch, page 111
- ☐ The Egg, page 112
- ☐ Quadriceps Stretch, page 113
- ☐ Hamstring Stretch, page 114
- ☐ Calf Stretch, page 115
- ☐ Butterfly Stretch, page 116

Mix It Up

You've made it through the Commitment Phase—congratulations! Walking is becoming a regular part of your life. Now's a good time to look back through your journal pages and see how far you've come.

Quote of the Day

Make no little plans; they have no magic to stir men's blood...Make big plans, aim high in hope and work.
—Daniel H. Burnham

209

Part 2
Walk the Weight Away!,
Day by Day

Nutrition Guide

If you've never tried sprouts, why not take the opportunity to give them a try. Sprouts add a delicious crunch to salads and sandwiches. Try a handful on your lunchtime ham sandwich. Sprouts are rich in protein and vitamins A, B complex, C, and E. In addition, they're good sources of various minerals and enzymes and low-cal too, with only 10 calories per cup.

Suggested Menu

Breakfast

3 frozen pancakes topped with 2 heaping tablespoons warmed applesauce

1 cup non-fat milk

Lunch

• 1 Chicken Salad Sandwich Italiano (page 55)

1 orange

1 handful pretzels

Dinner

• 1 piece Baked Chicken Siciliano (page 60)

¼ plate cooked rotini pasta with tomato sauce

1 small vegetable salad

2 shakes low-fat salad dressing

Snack

1 frozen fruit juice bar

210

Walk the **Weight Away!**

Breakfast time:
What I ate _____
_____
What I was doing while I ate
_____
Hunger level _____

Lunch time:
What I ate _____
_____
What I was doing while I ate
_____
Hunger level _____

Dinner time:
What I ate _____
_____
What I was doing while I ate
_____
Hunger level _____

Snack time:
What I ate _____
_____
What I was doing while I ate
_____
Hunger level _____

Water

Remember to drink 8 glasses of water

I feel ___ about how I ate today:

☐ satisfied

☐ proud

☐ disappointed

☐ other _____

My goals for tomorrow:

_____

_____

_____

Workout Journal

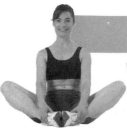

Pre-Walk Warm-Up

☐ **Spend 5 to 10 minutes slowly swinging your arms to prepare for your workout.**

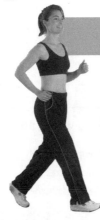

Walking Workout

Choose one.

☐ **Distance: 3 miles**
(15-minute-per-mile pace)

☐ **Time: 45 min.**
(15-minute-per-mile pace)

☐ **Steps: 6000 steps**

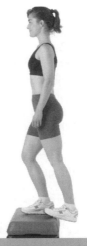

Strength Training

(1 set of 10 to 15 repetitions)

☐ **Shoulders Up,** page 118
☐ **Arm Power I,** page 119
☐ **Front Fly,** page 125
☐ **Push-Up,** page 124
☐ **Back Fly,** page 122
☐ **Thigh Shaper,** page 126
☐ **Best Butt,** page 127
☐ **Six Pack,** page 132
☐ **Basic Crunch,** page 133

Post-Walk Stretches

☐ **Neck Stretch,** page 107
☐ **Chest & Biceps Stretch,**
page 110
☐ **Triceps Stretch,** page 109
☐ **Upper Back Stretch,** page 111
☐ **Hamstring Stretch,** page 114
☐ **Quad Stretch,** page 113
☐ **Calf Stretch,** page 115

I feel __ about my workout today:

☐ satisfied
☐ proud
☐ disappointed
☐ other _____

My goals for tomorrow:

_____
_____
_____

Quote of the Day

What saves a man is to take a step. Then another step. It is always the same step, but you have to take it.
—Antoine de Saint-Exupery

Trainer's Tip

When you perform a squat, center your body weight over your heels rather than your toes. This will help you maintain good form.

211

Part 2
Walk the Weight Away!,
Day by Day

Nutrition Guide

Suggested Menu

Breakfast

½ large bagel

2 heaping teaspoons peanut butter

1 small box raisins

1 cup non-fat milk

Lunch

- 1 Brunch Wrap (page 47)

1 handful baby carrots

1 cup non-fat milk

Dinner

- 1 bowl Cheese Ravioli Soup (page 63)

1 small vegetable salad

2 shakes low-fat salad dressing

1 small dinner roll

1 teaspoon butter

Snack

1 cup fresh berries

Energy bars are a good source of quick energy when you need a lift, say in the middle of the day or just before a workout. But energy bars aren't necessarily low-fat or low-calorie. Many are loaded with sugar, and are some even packed with fat. So just as with any other food, it's important to read the label and choose wisely.

Breakfast   time:

What I ate _____

_____

What I was doing while I ate

_____

Hunger level _____

Lunch   time:

What I ate _____

_____

What I was doing while I ate

_____

Hunger level _____

Dinner   time:

What I ate _____

_____

What I was doing while I ate

_____

Hunger level _____

Snack   time:

What I ate _____

_____

What I was doing while I ate

_____

Hunger level _____

Water

Remember to drink 8 glasses of water

I feel ___ about how I ate today:

- ☐ satisfied
- ☐ proud
- ☐ disappointed
- ☐ other _____

My goals for tomorrow:

_____

_____

_____

212

Walk
the
Weight
Away!

Workout Journal

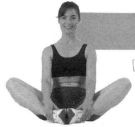

Pre-Walk Warm-Up

☐ **Spend 5 to 10 minutes slowly swinging your arms to prepare for your workout.**

Walking Workout

Choose one.

☐ **Distance: 3.5 miles**
(15-minute-per-mile pace)

☐ **Time: 53 min.**
(15-minute-per-mile pace)

☐ **Steps: 7000 steps**

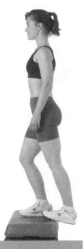

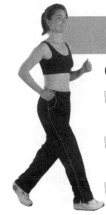

Strength Training

(2 set of 10 to 15 repetitions)
☐ **Arm Power II,** page 120
☐ **Tri Blaster,** page 121
☐ **Karate Kick,** page 128
☐ **Plié Press,** page 129
☐ **Hot Calves,** page 130
☐ **Strong Center,** page 131
☐ **Crunch Combo,** page 134

Post-Walk Stretches

☐ **Neck Stretch,** page 107
☐ **Chest & Biceps Stretch,** page 110
☐ **Triceps Stretch,** page 109
☐ **Upper Back Stretch,** page 111
☐ **Hamstring Stretch,** page 114
☐ **Quad Stretch,** page 113
☐ **Calf Stretch,** page 115

I feel ___ about my workout today:
☐ satisfied
☐ proud
☐ disappointed
☐ other _____

My goals for tomorrow:
_____
_____
_____

Quote of the Day
Opportunity is missed by most people because it is dressed in overalls and looks like work.
—Thomas A. Edison

Trainer's Tip
Taking pain relievers before a workout to prevent aches and pains is *not* a good idea. Products like aspirin and ibuprofen can cause stomach and intestinal distress.

213

Part 2
Walk the Weight Away!,
Day by Day

Nutrition Guide

Suggested Menu

Breakfast

½ large bagel

2 heaping teaspoons peanut butter

1 small box raisins

1 cup non-fat milk

Lunch

• Lemon Hummus Sandwich (page 57)

1 orange

Dinner

½ plate baked ham

¼ plate brown rice

• ¼ plate Cheesy Broccoli Gratin (page 83)

1 kiwifruit

Snack

½ baked potato with salsa

Next time you're craving ice cream, try low- or non-fat frozen yogurt or sorbet. Sometimes the craving is for something cold and sweet and those products just might do the trick.

Breakfast   time:

What I ate _____

_____

What I was doing while I ate

_____

Hunger level _____

Lunch   time:

What I ate _____

_____

What I was doing while I ate

_____

Hunger level _____

Dinner   time:

What I ate _____

_____

What I was doing while I ate

_____

Hunger level _____

Snack   time:

What I ate _____

_____

What I was doing while I ate

_____

Hunger level _____

Water

Remember to drink 8 glasses of water

I feel __ about how I ate today:

☐ satisfied

☐ proud

☐ disappointed

☐ other _____

My goals for tomorrow:

_____

_____

_____

214

Walk
the
Weight
Away!

Workout Journal

Daily Stretches

- ☐ Head & Neck Stretch, page 107
- ☐ Shoulder Stretch, page 108
- ☐ Triceps Stretch, page 109
- ☐ Chest & Biceps Stretch, page 110
- ☐ Upper Back Stretch, page 111
- ☐ The Egg, page 112
- ☐ Quadriceps Stretch, page 113
- ☐ Hamstring Stretch, page 114
- ☐ Calf Stretch, page 115
- ☐ Butterfly Stretch, page 116

An Elite Group

As a walker, you're in pretty good company. Some famous folks who were also avid walkers include Ralph Waldo Emerson, Henry David Thoreau, and presidents Jefferson, Lincoln, and Truman.

Breathe Easy

When people first take up exercise, they often worry about their breathing: Do I breathe through my mouth or my nose? The fact of the matter is that it doesn't matter. The important thing is to keep breathing.

Meet, But Don't Compete

When you walk with friends or family, don't turn the session into a race (unless that's what you want to do). Turning a workout into a competition can be discouraging or intimidating.

Quote of the Day

No one gets an iron-clad guarantee of success. Certainly, factors like opportunity, luck and timing are important. But the backbone of success is usually found in old fashioned, basic concepts like hard work, determination, good planning and perseverance.
—Merlin Olsen

215

Part 2
Walk the Weight Away!,
Day by Day

Nutrition Guide

Suggested Menu

Breakfast

2 slices whole-grain toast

2 teaspoons jam

½ pint scrambled egg sub-stitute, scrambled

½ grapefruit

Lunch

* 1 Veggie Pita Sandwich (page 59)

1 apple

1 handful nuts

Dinner

* 1 Oaty Beef Burger (page 63)

1 hamburger bun

1 small salad

2 shakes low-fat salad dressing

Snack

* 1 serving Grilled Pineapple Slices (page 85)

You're a little more than half way through the *Walk the Weight Away!* program. Take time to assess where you are and how you feel. Are you feeling satisfied with your eating habits? How much weight have you lost? Now might be a good time to take a mid-point photograph of yourself or to set up a graph that tracks your weight loss.

Breakfast   time:

What I ate _____

_____

What I was doing while I ate

_____

Hunger level _____

Lunch   time:

What I ate _____

_____

What I was doing while I ate

_____

Hunger level _____

Dinner   time:

What I ate _____

_____

What I was doing while I ate

_____

Hunger level _____

Snack   time:

What I ate _____

_____

What I was doing while I ate

_____

Hunger level _____

Water

Remember to drink 8 glasses of water

I feel ___ about how I ate today:

☐ satisfied

☐ proud

☐ disappointed

☐ other _____

My goals for tomorrow:

_____

_____

_____

Walk the **Weight** **Away!**

Workout Journal

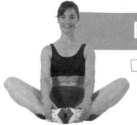

Pre-Walk Warm-Up

☐ Spend 5 to 10 minutes slowly swinging your arms to prepare for your workout.

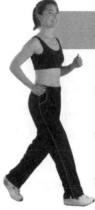

Walking Workout

Choose one.

☐ **Distance: 3.5 miles**
(15-minute-per-mile pace)

☐ **Time: 53 min.**
(15-minute-per-mile pace)

☐ **Steps: 7000 steps**

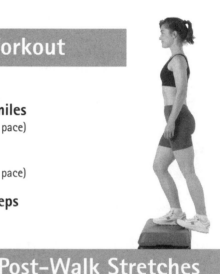

Strength Training

(2 set of 10 to 15 repetitions)

☐ **Shoulders Up,** page 118
☐ **Arm Power I,** page 119
☐ **Front Fly,** page 125
☐ **Push-Up,** page 124
☐ **Back Fly,** page 122
☐ **Thigh Shaper,** page 126
☐ **Best Butt,** page 127
☐ **Six Pack,** page 132
☐ **Basic Crunch,** page 133

Post-Walk Stretches

☐ **Neck Stretch,** page 107
☐ **Chest & Biceps Stretch,** page 110
☐ **Triceps Stretch,** page 109
☐ **Upper Back Stretch,** page 111
☐ **Hamstring Stretch,** page 114
☐ **Quad Stretch,** page 113
☐ **Calf Stretch,** page 115

I feel __ about my workout today:

☐ satisfied
☐ proud
☐ disappointed
☐ other _____

My goals for tomorrow:

_____

_____

_____

Quote of the Day
The gem cannot be polished without friction, nor man perfected without trials.
—Chinese Proverb

Trainer's Tip
Work different muscles by walking backward for a few paces now and then (don't lose your balance or bump into things). Walking forward works your glutes and calves; walking backward works your quadriceps and shin muscles.

217

Part 2
Walk the Weight Away!,
Day by Day

Nutrition Guide

Suggested Menu

Breakfast

1 bowl high-fiber cereal
1 cup non-fat milk
1 handful nuts

Lunch

- 1 plate Spinach Salad (page 90)
1 handful grapes
½ small whole grain bagel
1 teaspoon butter

Dinner

- 1 piece Grilled Marinated Salmon (page 70)
- ¼ plate Rice Pilaf (page 87)
- ½ plate Spinach Salad (page 90)

Snack

1 handful dried fruit

You may have heard that people who diet often or who "yo-yo" diet have a harder time losing weight. That's certainly a discouraging thought for those of us who have dieted before. But here's good news: A recent National Institutes of Health (NIH) study found that past dieting behaviors do *not* hurt your chances of success in the future. So just because you've tried and failed before doesn't mean you can't succeed now!

Breakfast   time:

What I ate _____

_____

What I was doing while I ate

_____

Hunger level _____

Lunch   time:

What I ate _____

_____

What I was doing while I ate

_____

Hunger level _____

Dinner   time:

What I ate _____

_____

What I was doing while I ate

_____

Hunger level _____

Snack   time:

What I ate _____

_____

What I was doing while I ate

_____

Hunger level _____

Water

Remember to drink 8 glasses of water

I feel ___ about how I ate today:

- [ ] satisfied
- [ ] proud
- [ ] disappointed
- [ ] other _____

My goals for tomorrow:

_____

_____

_____

218

Walk
the
Weight
Away!

Workout Journal

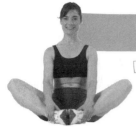

Pre-Walk Warm-Up

☐ **Spend 5 to 10 minutes slowly swinging your arms to prepare for your workout.**

Walking Workout

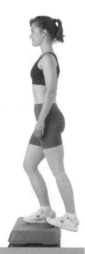

Choose one.

☐ **Distance: 3.5 miles**
(15-minute-per-mile pace)

☐ **Time: 53 min.**
(15-minute-per-mile pace)

☐ **Steps: 7000 steps**

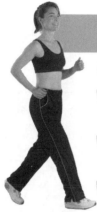

Strength Training

(2 set of 10 to 15 repetitions)

☐ **Arm Power II,** page 120
☐ **Tri Blaster,** page 121
☐ **Karate Kick,** page 128
☐ **Plié Press,** page 129
☐ **Hot Calves,** page 130
☐ **Strong Center,** page 131
☐ **Crunch Combo,** page 134

Post-Walk Stretches

☐ **Neck Stretch,** page 107
☐ **Chest & Biceps Stretch,** page 110
☐ **Triceps Stretch,** page 109
☐ **Upper Back Stretch,** page 111
☐ **Hamstring Stretch,** page 114
☐ **Quad Stretch,** page 113
☐ **Calf Stretch,** page 115

I feel ___ about my workout today:
☐ satisfied
☐ proud
☐ disappointed
☐ other _____

My goals for tomorrow:

_____

_____

_____

Quote of the Day
Do not anticipate trouble, or worry about what may never happen. Keep in the sunlight.
—Benjamin Franklin

Trainer's Tip
Your recovery heart-rate reading at the end of your workout, after you have cooled down, should be below your training zone. If it isn't, continue to cool down.

219

Part 2
Walk the Weight Away!,
Day by Day

Nutrition Guide

Suggested Menu

Breakfast

- 1 Graham Cracker Muffin
  (page 50)

  1 cup non-fat milk

  1 small banana

Lunch

- 1 Better-than-Pizza Potato
  (page 82)

  1 plum

Dinner

- 1 piece Baked
  Chicken Siciliano (page 60)

  ¼ plate cooked rotini pasta
  with tomato sauce

  1 small vegetable salad

  2 shakes low-fat
  salad dressing

Snack

1 frozen fruit juice bar

Nuts are a no-no when you're trying to lose weight, right? Not necessarily. Although nuts *do* have a high fat content, it's the healthy monosaturated fat that lowers cholesterol. They're also loaded with healthy nutrients. That makes nuts a satisfying, healthy indulgence in reasonable portion sizes.

Breakfast   time:

What I ate _____

_____

What I was doing while I ate

_____

Hunger level _____

Lunch   time:

What I ate _____

_____

What I was doing while I ate

_____

Hunger level _____

Dinner   time:

What I ate _____

_____

What I was doing while I ate

_____

Hunger level _____

Snack   time:

What I ate _____

_____

What I was doing while I ate

_____

Hunger level _____

Water

Remember to drink 8 glasses of water

I feel ___ about how I ate today:

- ☐ satisfied
- ☐ proud
- ☐ disappointed
- ☐ other _____

My goals for tomorrow:

_____

_____

_____

Walk the **Weight** Away!

Workout Journal

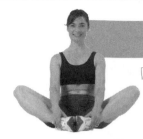

Pre-Walk Warm-Up

☐ Spend 5 to 10 minutes slowly swinging your arms to prepare for your workout.

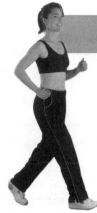

Walking Workout

Choose one.

☐ **Distance: 3.5 miles**
(15-minute-per-mile pace)

☐ **Time: 53 min.**
(15-minute-per-mile pace)

☐ **Steps: 7000 steps**

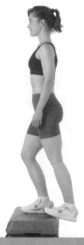

Strength Training

(1 set of 10 to 15 repetitions)

☐ **Shoulders Up,** page 118
☐ **Arm Power I,** page 119
☐ **Front Fly,** page 125
☐ **Push-Up,** page 124
☐ **Back Fly,** page 122
☐ **Thigh Shaper,** page 126
☐ **Best Butt,** page 127
☐ **Six Pack,** page 132
☐ **Basic Crunch,** page 133

Post-Walk Stretches

☐ **Neck Stretch,** page 107
☐ **Chest & Biceps Stretch,** page 110
☐ **Triceps Stretch,** page 109
☐ **Upper Back Stretch,** page 111
☐ **Hamstring Stretch,** page 114
☐ **Quad Stretch,** page 113
☐ **Calf Stretch,** page 115

I feel ___ about my workout today:

☐ satisfied
☐ proud
☐ disappointed
☐ other _____

My goals for tomorrow:

_____

_____

_____

Quote of the Day
Cheerfulness keeps up a kind of daylight in the mind, filling it with a steady and perpetual serenity.
—Joseph Addison

Trainer's Tip
If you ever feel dizzy when exercising slow down, and gradually come to a stop. Don't suddenly stop moving entirely.

221

Part 2
Walk the Weight Away!,
Day by Day

Nutrition Guide

Suggested Menu

Breakfast

- 2 slices French Toast (page 49)

  1 orange

1 slice Canadian bacon

Lunch

- 1 Strawberry Orange Muffin (page 52)

  1 apple

1 small container non-fat, no sugar added yogurt

Dinner

- 1 Kielbasa Kebab (page 71)

  1 small baked potato

  1 small salad

  2 shakes non-fat salad dressing

Snack

- 1 teaspoon peanut butter and 3 crackers

222

Walk
the
Weight
Away!

In winter, fresh fruit isn't nearly as plentiful as in warm weather. That's when dried fruit can provide a healthy, satisfying nutrient-rich alternative. Raisins, apricots, dates, and cherries (among others) are all delicious in pancake batters, and on muffins and cereal. Dried fruit is, in general, higher in calories than fresh fruit, so pay attention to portion sizes.

Breakfast   time:

What I ate _____

_____

What I was doing while I ate

_____

Hunger level _____

Lunch   time:

What I ate _____

_____

What I was doing while I ate

_____

Hunger level _____

Dinner   time:

What I ate _____

_____

What I was doing while I ate

_____

Hunger level _____

Snack   time:

What I ate _____

_____

What I was doing while I ate

_____

Hunger level _____

Water

Remember to drink 8 glasses of water

I feel ___ about how I ate today:

☐ satisfied

☐ proud

☐ disappointed

☐ other _____

My goals for tomorrow:

_____

_____

_____

Workout Journal

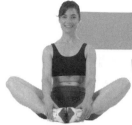

Pre-Walk Warm-Up

☐ **Spend 5 to 10 minutes slowly swinging your arms to prepare for your workout.**

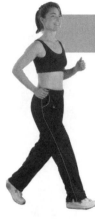

Walking Workout

Choose one.

☐ **Distance: 3.5 miles**
(15-minute-per-mile pace)

☐ **Time: 53 min.**
(15-minute-per-mile pace)

☐ **Steps: 7000 steps**

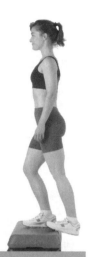

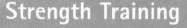

Strength Training

(3 set of 10 to 15 repetitions)

☐ **Arm Power II,** page 120
☐ **Tri Blaster,** page 121
☐ **Karate Kick,** page 128
☐ **Plié Press,** page 129
☐ **Hot Calves,** page 130
☐ **Strong Center,** page 131
☐ **Crunch Combo,** page 134

Post-Walk Stretches

☐ **Neck Stretch,** page 107
☐ **Chest & Biceps Stretch,** page 110
☐ **Triceps Stretch,** page 109
☐ **Upper Back Stretch,** page 111
☐ **Hamstring Stretch,** page 114
☐ **Quad Stretch,** page 113
☐ **Calf Stretch,** page 115

I feel __ about my workout today:
☐ satisfied
☐ proud
☐ disappointed
☐ other _____

My goals for tomorrow:

_____

_____

_____

Quote of the Day

Experience is not what happens to you; it's what you do with what happens to you.
—Aldous Huxley

Trainer's Tip

If you have only 15 minutes on a given day to devote to your walk, go ahead anyway. It is important that your workouts are consistent and regular.

223

Part 2
Walk the Weight Away!,
Day by Day

Nutrition Guide

Suggested Menu

Breakfast

- 1 Cheesy Potato Omelette (page 48)

  1 slice whole wheat toast with 1 teaspoon butter

  ¼ cantaloupe

Lunch

- 1 cup Chicken & Sundried Tomato Pasta Salad (page 64)

  1 cup non-fat milk

  1 orange

Dinner

- 1 bowl Spunky Vegetarian Chili (page 79)

  4 saltines

  1 small plate vegetable salad

  2 shakes low-fat salad dressing

Snack

2 large graham crackers

224

Walk
the
Weight
Away!

Fruit juice can be part of a healthful diet, but make sure that the juice you're drinking is not loaded with added sugar. Many juices (including some brands of cranberry, for instance) have as much as 70 percent added sugar. Your best bet? Choose juices that are labeled "100 percent real fruit juice."

Breakfast   time:

What I ate _____

_____

What I was doing while I ate

_____

Hunger level _____

Lunch   time:

What I ate _____

_____

What I was doing while I ate

_____

Hunger level _____

Dinner   time:

What I ate _____

_____

What I was doing while I ate

_____

Hunger level _____

Snack   time:

What I ate _____

_____

What I was doing while I ate

_____

Hunger level _____

Water

Remember to drink 8 glasses of water

I feel ___ about how I ate today:

☐ satisfied

☐ proud

☐ disappointed

☐ other _____

My goals for tomorrow:

_____

_____

_____

Workout Journal

Daily Stretches

- ☐ Head & Neck Stretch, page 107
- ☐ Shoulder Stretch, page 108
- ☐ Triceps Stretch, page 109
- ☐ Chest & Biceps Stretch, page 110
- ☐ Upper Back Stretch, page 111

- ☐ The Egg, page 112
- ☐ Quadriceps Stretch, page 113
- ☐ Hamstring Stretch, page 114
- ☐ Calf Stretch, page 115
- ☐ Butterfly Stretch, page 116

Become an Award Winner

Now that you're walking regularly, you can win an award—the Presidential Sports Award. To find out how, log onto www.fitness.gov/sports/sports.html

How Far You've Come

Have you been adding up your mileage, time, or steps? Now's a good time to tally your results.

Enter a Race

Who says races are just for runners? Plenty of races welcome and even encourage walkers to enter. The Revlon Run/Walk for Women is one such event. To find others, visit your local recreation center, track, or YMCA, which usually have postings for such events.

Quote of the Day

Behold the turtle. He makes progress only when he sticks his neck out.

—James Bryant Conant

225

Part 2
Walk the Weight Away!,
Day by Day

Nutrition Guide

Suggested Menu

Breakfast

½ large bagel

2 heaping teaspoons peanut butter

1 small box raisins

1 cup non-fat milk

Lunch

- 1 Brunch Wrap (page 47)

1 handful baby carrots

1 cup non-fat milk

Dinner

- 1 bowl Cheese Ravioli Soup (page 63)

1 small vegetable salad

2 shakes low-fat salad dressing

1 small dinner roll

1 teaspoon butter

Snack

1 handful pretzels

226

Walk the **Weight Away!**

When grilling season rolls around, take advantage of the bounty of fresh vegetables by making kebabs. Marinate chunks of zucchini, mushrooms, and red and green pepper in low- or non-fat vinaigrette for at least 2 hours. Thread the vegetable chunks onto skewers and grill until tender. They're easy to make, delicious, low-fat, and healthful.

Breakfast   time:

What I ate _____

_____

What I was doing while I ate

_____

Hunger level _____

Lunch   time:

What I ate _____

_____

What I was doing while I ate

_____

Hunger level _____

Dinner   time:

What I ate _____

_____

What I was doing while I ate

_____

Hunger level _____

Snack   time:

What I ate _____

_____

What I was doing while I ate

_____

Hunger level _____

Water

Remember to drink 8 glasses of water

I feel ___ about how I ate today:

☐ satisfied

☐ proud

☐ disappointed

☐ other _____

My goals for tomorrow:

_____

_____

_____

Workout Journal

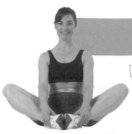

Pre-Walk Warm-Up

☐ **Spend 5 to 10 minutes slowly swinging your arms to prepare for your workout.**

Walking Workout

Choose one.

☐ **Distance: 3.5 miles**
(15-minute-per-mile pace)

☐ **Time: 42 min.**
(15-minute-per-mile pace)

☐ **Steps: 7000 steps**

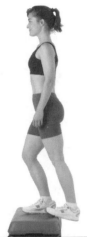

Strength Training

(3 set of 10 to 15 repetitions)

☐ **Shoulders Up,** page 118
☐ **Arm Power I,** page 119
☐ **Front Fly,** page 125
☐ **Push-Up,** page 124
☐ **Back Fly,** page 122
☐ **Thigh Shaper,** page 126
☐ **Best Butt,** page 127
☐ **Six Pack,** page 132
☐ **Basic Crunch,** page 133

Post-Walk Stretches

☐ **Neck Stretch,** page 107
☐ **Chest & Biceps Stretch,** page 110
☐ **Triceps Stretch,** page 109
☐ **Upper Back Stretch,** page 111
☐ **Hamstring Stretch,** page 114
☐ **Quad Stretch,** page 113
☐ **Calf Stretch,** page 115

I feel ___ about my workout today:

☐ satisfied
☐ proud
☐ disappointed
☐ other _____

My goals for tomorrow:

_____

_____

_____

Quote of the Day
Courage is the ladder on which all the other virtues mount.
—Clare Booth Luce

Trainer's Tip
If you feel irritable, experience insomnia, get injured, or frequently come down with colds, you may be overtraining. Don't ignore these signs; tone down the intensity of your workout.

227

Part 2
Walk the Weight Away!,
Day by Day

Nutrition Guide

Suggested Menu

Breakfast

3 frozen pancakes topped with 2 heaping tablespoons warmed applesauce

1 cup non-fat milk

Lunch

- 1 small plate Waldorf Salad (page 92)

4 saltines

Dinner

- 1 piece Baked Chicken Siciliano (page 60)

¼ plate cooked rotini pasta with tomato sauce

1 small vegetable salad

2 shakes low-fat salad dressing

Snack

½ small bagel with jam

Today's breakfast menu calls for warmed applesauce. Many commercial brands are loaded with sugar, so why not make your own? It's quick and easy. Peel one or two apples—any kinds you like—and cut them into chunks. Place them, with a little water, in a small saucepan. Warm the apples over low heat until they soften and become applesauce. If you like, you can jazz them up with a little cinnamon or a pinch of ground cloves.

Breakfast   time:

What I ate _____

_____

What I was doing while I ate

_____

Hunger level _____

Lunch   time:

What I ate _____

_____

What I was doing while I ate

_____

Hunger level _____

Dinner   time:

What I ate _____

_____

What I was doing while I ate

_____

Hunger level _____

Snack   time:

What I ate _____

_____

What I was doing while I ate

_____

Hunger level _____

228

Water

Remember to drink 8 glasses of water

I feel __ about how I ate today:

- ☐ satisfied
- ☐ proud
- ☐ disappointed
- ☐ other _____

My goals for tomorrow:

_____

_____

_____

Walk the **Weight** **Away!**

Workout Journal

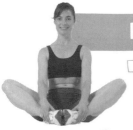

Pre-Walk Warm-Up

☐ Spend 5 to 10 minutes slowly swinging your arms to prepare for your workout.

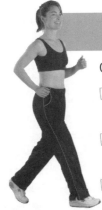

Walking Workout

Choose one.

☐ **Distance: 3.5 miles**
(12-minute-per-mile pace)

☐ **Time: 42 min.**
(12-minute-per-mile pace)

☐ **Steps: 7000 steps**

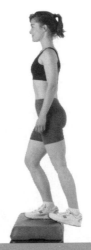

Strength Training

(3 set of 10 to 15 repetitions)

☐ **Arm Power II**, page 120
☐ **Tri Blaster**, page 121
☐ **Karate Kick**, page 128
☐ **Plié Press**, page 129
☐ **Hot Calves**, page 130
☐ **Strong Center**, page 131
☐ **Crunch Combo**, page 134

Post-Walk Stretches

☐ **Neck Stretch**, page 107
☐ **Chest & Biceps Stretch**, page 110
☐ **Triceps Stretch**, page 109
☐ **Upper Back Stretch**, page 111
☐ **Hamstring Stretch**, page 114
☐ **Quad Stretch**, page 113
☐ **Calf Stretch**, page 115

Quote of the Day

Aerodynamically, the bumble bee shouldn't be able to fly, but the bumble bee doesn't know it so it goes on flying anyway.
—Mary Kay Ash

Trainer's Tip

Did you know you can be thin and fat at the same time? Use a skin fold caliper to check your body fat percentage and find out whether your weight is comprised primarily of lean mass or fat.

229

I feel __ about my workout today:

☐ satisfied
☐ proud
☐ disappointed
☐ other _____

My goals for tomorrow:

_____

_____

_____

Part 2
Walk the Weight Away!,
Day by Day

Nutrition Guide

Suggested Menu

Breakfast

1 small container non-fat yogurt mixed with 2 heaping tablespoons Grapenuts cereal

1 cup grapefruit juice

Lunch

- 1 Veggie Pita Sandwich (page 59)

1 apple

1 handful nuts

Dinner

- 1 piece Buttery Almond Fish (page 62)

¼ plate brown rice

½ plate broccoli

1 cup non-fat milk

Snack

2 handfuls popcorn or 2 rice cakes

230

Walk the **Weight Away!**

Next time you crave a hamburger, why not try a veggie burger? There are so many varieties available you're sure to find one that you like. Worried it'll taste like cardboard? Unlike some of the "fake" burgers of years ago, today's brands are delicious. Most brands cook up in the microwave, so they're a good lunch option, too.

Breakfast   time:

What I ate _____

_____

What I was doing while I ate

_____

Hunger level _____

Lunch   time:

What I ate _____

_____

What I was doing while I ate

_____

Hunger level _____

Dinner   time:

What I ate _____

_____

What I was doing while I ate

_____

Hunger level _____

Snack   time:

What I ate _____

_____

What I was doing while I ate

_____

Hunger level _____

Water

Remember to drink 8 glasses of water

I feel ___ about how I ate today:

☐ satisfied

☐ proud

☐ disappointed

☐ other _____

My goals for tomorrow:

_____

_____

_____

Workout Journal

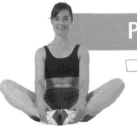

Pre-Walk Warm-Up

☐ Spend 5 to 10 minutes slowly swinging your arms to prepare for your workout.

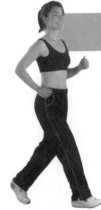

Walking Workout

Choose one.

☐ **Distance: 3.5 miles**
(12-minute-per-mile pace)

☐ **Time: 42 min.**
(12-minute-per-mile pace)

☐ **Steps: 7000 steps**

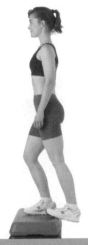

Strength Training

(3 set of 10 to 15 repetitions)

☐ **Shoulders Up,** page 118
☐ **Arm Power I,** page 119
☐ **Front Fly,** page 125
☐ **Push-Up,** page 124
☐ **Back Fly,** page 122
☐ **Thigh Shaper,** page 126
☐ **Best Butt,** page 127
☐ **Six Pack,** page 132
☐ **Basic Crunch,** page 133

Post-Walk Stretches

☐ **Neck Stretch,** page 107
☐ **Chest & Biceps Stretch,** page 110
☐ **Triceps Stretch,** page 109
☐ **Upper Back Stretch,** page 111
☐ **Hamstring Stretch,** page 114
☐ **Quad Stretch,** page 113
☐ **Calf Stretch,** page 115

I feel __ about my workout today:

☐ satisfied
☐ proud
☐ disappointed
☐ other _____

My goals for tomorrow:

_____

_____

_____

Quote of the Day

No pessimist ever discovered the secret of the stars, or sailed to an uncharted land, or opened a new doorway for the human spirit.
—Helen Keller

Trainer's Tip

Never measure your body fat after you've been working out; the results will be skewed.

231

Part 2
Walk the Weight Away!,
Day by Day

Nutrition Guide

Suggested Menu

Breakfast

1 bowl high-fiber cereal

1 cup non-fat milk

1 handful nuts

Lunch

• 2 slices Pizza Primavera
(page 73)

1 orange

1 handful pretzels

Dinner

• 1 ½ cups Thai Pasta Salad
(page 91)

1 small plate mixed berries

1 small dinner roll

1 teaspoon butter

Snack

1 low-fat bran muffin

When you're at a party, it's easy to lose sight of your weight loss goals, especially after a few cocktails. Alcohol not only increases your appetite, it also lowers your resistance—and that can lead to overeating. If you want to be part of the celebration but skip the alcohol, there are several options: Sparkling cider has the bubbles of champagne, but none of the alcohol. Seltzer with lemon or lime is a no-calorie alternative to a cocktail, too.

Breakfast   time:

What I ate _____

_____

What I was doing while I ate

_____

Hunger level _____

Lunch   time:

What I ate _____

_____

What I was doing while I ate

_____

Hunger level _____

Dinner   time:

What I ate _____

_____

What I was doing while I ate

_____

Hunger level _____

Snack   time:

What I ate _____

_____

What I was doing while I ate

_____

Hunger level _____

Water

Remember to drink 8 glasses of water

I feel ___ about how I ate today:

☐ satisfied

☐ proud

☐ disappointed

☐ other _____

My goals for tomorrow:

_____

_____

232

Walk
the
Weight
Away!

Workout Journal

Daily Stretches

- ☐ Head & Neck Stretch, page 107
- ☐ Shoulder Stretch, page 108
- ☐ Triceps Stretch, page 109
- ☐ Chest & Biceps Stretch, page 110
- ☐ Upper Back Stretch, page 111

- ☐ The Egg, page 112
- ☐ Quadriceps Stretch, page 113
- ☐ Hamstring Stretch, page 114
- ☐ Calf Stretch, page 115
- ☐ Butterfly Stretch, page 116

Take a Break

 Anytime you feel that you're having trouble keeping up with the walking schedule, go ahead and back up a week or two. There's no harm and you'll benefit from not wearing yourself out in the long run.

Miss a Week? Don't Panic

You've been following the *Walk the Weight Away!* Plan for six weeks now. But what happens if you miss a week because of illness (or any other reason)? Don't worry; you won't lose your level of fitness. When you're ready to begin again, repeat the week you left off at, then continue as you were.

Time for New Shoes?

If you're like many people, you wear a pair of shoes until they're falling apart. But don't take that approach with your walking shoes. A good rule of thumb is to replace them every 300 miles (yet another reason to keep up with your workout journal).

Quote of the Day
A will finds a way.
—Orison Swett Marden

233

Part 2
Walk the Weight Away!,
Day by Day

Nutrition Guide

Suggested Menu

Breakfast

2 slices whole-grain toast

2 teaspoons jam

½ pint egg substitute, scrambled

½ grapefruit

Lunch

- 1 plate Spinach Salad (page 90)

1 handful grapes

½ small whole grain bagel

1 teaspoon butter

Dinner

- 1 piece Crispy Chicken (page 69)
- ¼ plate Smashed Potatoes (page 89)
- ½ plate Nutty Balsamic Green Beans (page 86)

1 individual container applesauce

Snack

1 frozen fruit juice bar

234

Walk the Weight Away!

One way some people keep from snacking is by brushing their teeth immediately after every meal. When your mouth is freshly brushed and feels clean, suddenly eating doesn't seem like such a good idea. So not only are you suppressing your appetite, you're doing something good for your dental health.

Breakfast   time:

What I ate _____

_____

What I was doing while I ate

_____

Hunger level _____

Lunch   time:

What I ate _____

_____

What I was doing while I ate

_____

Hunger level _____

Dinner   time:

What I ate _____

_____

What I was doing while I ate

_____

Hunger level _____

Snack   time:

What I ate _____

_____

What I was doing while I ate

_____

Hunger level _____

Water

Remember to drink 8 glasses of water

I feel ___ about how I ate today:

- ☐ satisfied
- ☐ proud
- ☐ disappointed
- ☐ other _____

My goals for tomorrow:

_____

_____

_____

Workout Journal

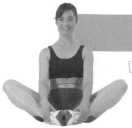

Pre-Walk Warm-Up

☐ **Spend 5 to 10 minutes slowly swinging your arms to prepare for your workout.**

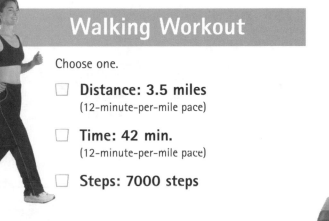

Walking Workout

Choose one.

☐ **Distance: 3.5 miles**
(12-minute-per-mile pace)

☐ **Time: 42 min.**
(12-minute-per-mile pace)

☐ **Steps: 7000 steps**

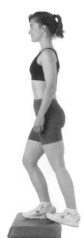

Strength Training

(3 set of 10 to 15 repetitions)

☐ **Arm Power II**, page 120
☐ **Tri Blaster**, page 121
☐ **Karate Kick**, page 128
☐ **Plié Press**, page 129
☐ **Hot Calves**, page 130
☐ **Strong Center**, page 131
☐ **Crunch Combo**, page 134

Post-Walk Stretches

☐ **Neck Stretch**, page 107
☐ **Chest & Biceps Stretch**, page 110
☐ **Triceps Stretch**, page 109
☐ **Upper Back Stretch**, page 111
☐ **Hamstring Stretch**, page 114
☐ **Quad Stretch**, page 113
☐ **Calf Stretch**, page 115

Quote of the Day
It's always too early to quit.
—Norman Vincent Peale

Trainer's Tip
To determine your resting heart rate, measure your heart rate first thing in the morning before you get out of bed. Lower resting heart rates usually correspond with higher levels of fitness. Higher rates can indicate overtraining.

I feel ___ about my workout today:
☐ satisfied
☐ proud
☐ disappointed
☐ other _____

My goals for tomorrow:
_____
_____
_____

235

Part 2
Walk the Weight Away!, **Day by Day**

Nutrition Guide

Suggested Menu

Breakfast

- 1 Greek Omelette
  (page 51)
- ½ English muffin
- 1 teaspoon jam
- 1 cup berries

Lunch

- 1 plate Spinach Salad
  (page 90)
- 1 handful grapes
- ½ small whole grain bagel
- 1 teaspoon butter

Dinner

- ¾ cup Barbecued Pork
  (page 61)
- 1 whole grain
  hamburger bun
- 1 cup vegetable salad
- 1 small watermelon wedge

Snack

- 1 piece fresh fruit

There are several elements that make food appealing: aroma, flavor, and appearance. Don't neglect how your food looks when you prepare and serve it. When food smells good and looks appetizing, it tastes better and is more satisfying. Chefs call it "presentation."

Use your imagination when serving food. Arrange it neatly on the plate; use garnishes such as fruit wedges; experiment with interesting serving dishes, like serving fruit salad or frozen yogurt in a champagne or wine glass.

Breakfast   time:

What I ate _____

_____

What I was doing while I ate

_____

Hunger level _____

Lunch   time:

What I ate _____

_____

What I was doing while I ate

_____

Hunger level _____

Dinner   time:

What I ate _____

_____

What I was doing while I ate

_____

Hunger level _____

Snack   time:

What I ate _____

_____

What I was doing while I ate

_____

Hunger level _____

Water

Remember to drink 8 glasses of water

I feel ___ about how I ate today:

- ☐ satisfied
- ☐ proud
- ☐ disappointed
- ☐ other _____

My goals for tomorrow:

_____

_____

_____

236

Walk
the
Weight
Away!

Workout Journal

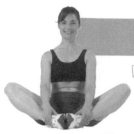

Pre-Walk Warm-Up

☐ **Spend 5 to 10 minutes slowly swinging your arms to prepare for your workout.**

Walking Workout

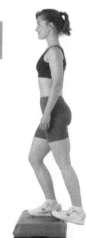

Choose one.

☐ **Distance: 3.5 miles**
(12-minute-per-mile pace)

☐ **Time: 42 min.**
(12-minute-per-mile pace)

☐ **Steps: 7000 steps**

Strength Training

(3 set of 10 to 15 repetitions)

☐ **Shoulders Up,** page 118
☐ **Arm Power I,** page 119
☐ **Front Fly,** page 125
☐ **Push-Up,** page 124
☐ **Back Fly,** page 122
☐ **Thigh Shaper,** page 126
☐ **Best Butt,** page 127
☐ **Six Pack,** page 132
☐ **Basic Crunch,** page 133

Post-Walk Stretches

☐ **Neck Stretch,** page 107
☐ **Chest & Biceps Stretch,** page 110
☐ **Triceps Stretch,** page 109
☐ **Upper Back Stretch,** page 111
☐ **Hamstring Stretch,** page 114
☐ **Quad Stretch,** page 113
☐ **Calf Stretch,** page 115

I feel ___ about my workout today:

☐ satisfied
☐ proud
☐ disappointed
☐ other _____

My goals for tomorrow:

_____

_____

_____

Quote of the Day
Every exit is an entry somewhere.
—Tom Stoppard

Trainer's Tip
For longer walks you may want to wear a small backpack to carry your water and maybe a jacket. Just be careful not to load it up. A pack that's too heavy can change your gait and lead to injury.

237

Part 2
Walk the Weight Away!,
Day by Day

Nutrition Guide

Suggested Menu

Breakfast

- 1 Blueberry Muffin (page 46)

    1 small banana

    1 cup non-fat milk

Lunch

- 1 Better-than-Pizza Potato (page 82)

    1 Orange

    1 handful pretzels

Dinner

- 1 piece Grilled Marinated Salmon (page 70)
  - ¼ plate Rice Pilaf (page 87)
  - ½ plate Spinach Salad (page 90)

Snack

½ small bagel with jam

238

Walk
the
Weight
Away!

Prepackaged foods like deli meat and cheese save time, but they don't always save calories. Packaged cheese and meats usually come in 1-ounce slices, which may be more than you really need or want. A better idea is to buy those products from the store's deli counter, asking that they be sliced thin.

Breakfast   time:

What I ate _____

_____

What I was doing while I ate

_____

Hunger level _____

Lunch   time:

What I ate _____

_____

What I was doing while I ate

_____

Hunger level _____

Dinner   time:

What I ate _____

_____

What I was doing while I ate

_____

Hunger level _____

Snack   time:

What I ate _____

_____

What I was doing while I ate

_____

Hunger level _____

Water

Remember to drink 8 glasses of water

I feel __ about how I ate today:

- ☐ satisfied
- ☐ proud
- ☐ disappointed
- ☐ other _____

My goals for tomorrow:

_____

_____

_____

Workout Journal

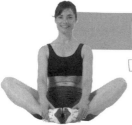

Pre-Walk Warm-Up

☐ **Spend 5 to 10 minutes slowly swinging your arms to prepare for your workout.**

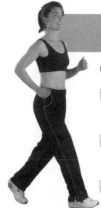

Walking Workout

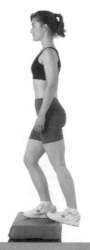

Choose one.

☐ **Distance: 3.5 miles**
(12-minute-per-mile pace)

☐ **Time: 42 min.**
(12-minute-per-mile pace)

☐ **Steps: 7000 steps**

Strength Training

(3 set of 10 to 15 repetitions)
☐ **Arm Power II,** page 120
☐ **Tri Blaster,** page 121
☐ **Karate Kick,** page 128
☐ **Plié Press,** page 129
☐ **Hot Calves,** page 130
☐ **Strong Center,** page 131
☐ **Crunch Combo,** page 134

Post-Walk Stretches

☐ **Neck Stretch,** page 107
☐ **Chest & Biceps Stretch,** page 110
☐ **Triceps Stretch,** page 109
☐ **Upper Back Stretch,** page 111
☐ **Hamstring Stretch,** page 114
☐ **Quad Stretch,** page 113
☐ **Calf Stretch,** page 115

Quote of the Day
It's always helpful to learn from your mistakes because then your mistakes seem worthwhile.
—Garry Marshall

Trainer's Tip
When doing abdominal exercises, try not to pull on your head or neck. You should be able to fit a fist between your chin and your chest.

239

I feel __ about my workout today:
☐ satisfied
☐ proud
☐ disappointed
☐ other _____

My goals for tomorrow:
_____
_____
_____

Part 2
Walk the Weight Away!,
Day by Day

Nutrition Guide

Suggested Menu

Breakfast

1 bowl high-fiber cereal

1 cup non-fat milk

1 handful nuts

Lunch

• 1 Strawberry Orange Muffin (page 52)

1 apple

1 small container non-fat, no sugar added yogurt

Dinner

• 1 piece Baked Chicken Siciliano (page 60)

¼ plate cooked rotini pasta with tomato sauce

1 small vegetable salad

2 shakes low-fat salad dressing

Snack

1 handful Teddy Grahams

Soups made of broth and vegetables are delicious and make healthful lunches and dinners. But sometimes (especially during the colder months) those thin soups need a little oomph. There are several ways to thicken soup without cream or other high-fat additives. The first is by adding mashed potato flakes. Just stir a couple of tablespoons into the broth. A second is to add additional cooked and pureed vegetables into the broth.

Breakfast   time:

What I ate _____

_____

What I was doing while I ate

_____

Hunger level _____

Lunch   time:

What I ate _____

_____

What I was doing while I ate

_____

Hunger level _____

Dinner   time:

What I ate _____

_____

What I was doing while I ate

_____

Hunger level _____

Snack   time:

What I ate _____

_____

What I was doing while I ate

_____

Hunger level _____

Water

Remember to drink 8 glasses of water

I feel ___ about how I ate today:

☐ satisfied

☐ proud

☐ disappointed

☐ other _____

My goals for tomorrow:

_____

_____

_____

240

Walk the **Weight** **Away!**

Workout Journal

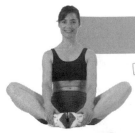

Pre-Walk Warm-Up

☐ Spend 5 to 10 minutes slowly swinging your arms to prepare for your workout.

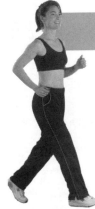

Walking Workout

Choose one.

☐ **Distance: 3.5 miles**
(12-minute-per-mile pace)

☐ **Time: 42 min.**
(12-minute-per-mile pace)

☐ **Steps: 7000 steps**

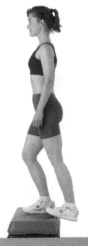

Strength Training

(3 set of 10 to 15 repetitions)
☐ **Shoulders Up,** page 118
☐ **Arm Power I,** page 119
☐ **Front Fly,** page 125
☐ **Push-Up,** page 124
☐ **Back Fly,** page 122
☐ **Thigh Shaper,** page 126
☐ **Best Butt,** page 127
☐ **Six Pack,** page 132
☐ **Basic Crunch,** page 133

Post-Walk Stretches

☐ **Neck Stretch,** page 107
☐ **Chest & Biceps Stretch,** page 110
☐ **Triceps Stretch,** page 109
☐ **Upper Back Stretch,** page 111
☐ **Hamstring Stretch,** page 114
☐ **Quad Stretch,** page 113
☐ **Calf Stretch,** page 115

Quote of the Day
Courage is not the absence of fear, but rather the judgment that something else is more important than fear.
—Ambrose Redmoon

Trainer's Tip
Walking in a mall is great in bad weather. Just make sure you don't stop to look in all the store windows—keep moving!

241

I feel ___ about my workout today:
☐ satisfied
☐ proud
☐ disappointed
☐ other _____

My goals for tomorrow:
_____
_____
_____

Part 2
Walk the Weight Away!,
Day by Day

Date:

Nutrition Guide

Suggested Menu

Breakfast
- 1 Graham Cracker Muffin (page 50)
  - 1 cup non-fat milk
  - 1 small banana

Lunch
- 1 ½ cups Thai Pasta Salad (page 91)
  - 1 pear

Dinner
- 1 piece Citrus Orange Roughy (page 68)
  - ¼ plate brown rice
  - ¼ plate peas
  - ¼ cantaloupe

Snack
1 handful steamed shrimp sprinkled with lemon juice and Old Bay seasoning

242

Walk the **Weight Away!**

Heard of so-called negative-calorie foods? They're foods—such as celery—that have so few calories that you actually lose weight chewing and digesting them. Unfortunately, negative-calorie foods are a dieting myth. While celery certainly is crunchy and refreshing, you won't melt away the pounds by eating it.

Breakfast   time:
What I ate _____

_____

What I was doing while I ate

_____

Hunger level _____

Lunch   time:
What I ate _____

_____

What I was doing while I ate

_____

Hunger level _____

Dinner   time:
What I ate _____

_____

What I was doing while I ate

_____

Hunger level _____

Snack   time:
What I ate _____

_____

What I was doing while I ate

_____

Hunger level _____

Water
Remember to drink 8 glasses of water

I feel __ about how I ate today:
- ☐ satisfied
- ☐ proud
- ☐ disappointed
- ☐ other _____

My goals for tomorrow:

_____

_____

_____

Workout Journal

Daily Stretches

☐ Head & Neck Stretch, page 107

☐ Shoulder Stretch, page 108

☐ Triceps Stretch, page 109

☐ Chest & Biceps Stretch, page 110

☐ Upper Back Stretch, page 111

☐ The Egg, page 112

☐ Quadriceps Stretch, page 113

☐ Hamstring Stretch, page 114

☐ Calf Stretch, page 115

☐ Butterfly Stretch, page 116

Quote of the Day
If you don't try, you've already failed.
—Anonymous

Workout Sniffles

You have a cold. Is it okay to workout? As long as that cold is restricted to your nose and throat, go ahead. But if it's moved into your chest, best to give it a rest for a day or two.

Breathe Easier

An anti-snoring device may help your workout: Many athletes swear by nasal strips, adhesive bands that you place across your nose. They open your nostrils, which not only reduces snoring, but makes it easier to breathe during your workout. The strips are sold in drugstores.

TV Time

Try doing your daily stretching routine as you watch your favorite evening television show

243

Part 2
*Walk the
Weight Away!*,
Day by Day

Nutrition Guide

Suggested Menu

Breakfast

2 slices whole-grain toast

2 teaspoons jam

½ pint scrambled egg substitute, scrambled

½ grapefruit

Lunch

• 1 Veggie Pita Sandwich (page 59)

1 apple

1 handful nuts

Dinner

1 low-fat hotdog

1 hotdog roll

1 handful low-fat chips

¼ plate baked beans

Snack

1 handful pretzels

Most Americans don't get anywhere near the recommended 20 to 35 grams of fiber in their diets, and that's too bad, because fiber reduces the risk of type 2 diabetes and heart disease. Not only that, but high fiber foods make you feel fuller, longer. To boost your fiber intake, eat more beans, brown rice, whole wheat bread, and vegetables.

Breakfast   time:

What I ate _____

_____

What I was doing while I ate

_____

Hunger level _____

Lunch   time:

What I ate _____

_____

What I was doing while I ate

_____

Hunger level _____

Dinner   time:

What I ate _____

_____

What I was doing while I ate

_____

Hunger level _____

Snack   time:

What I ate _____

_____

What I was doing while I ate

_____

Hunger level _____

Water

Remember to drink 8 glasses of water

I feel ___ about how I ate today:

☐ satisfied

☐ proud

☐ disappointed

☐ other _____

My goals for tomorrow:

_____

_____

_____

244

Walk the Weight Away!

Workout Journal

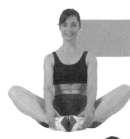

Pre-Walk Warm-Up

☐ Spend 5 to 10 minutes slowly swinging your arms to prepare for your workout.

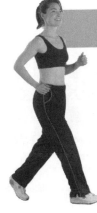

Walking Workout

Choose one.

☐ **Distance: 3.5 miles**
(12-minute-per-mile pace)

☐ **Time: 42 min.**
(12-minute-per-mile pace)

☐ **Steps: 7000 steps**

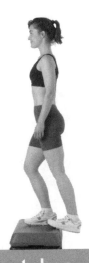

Strength Training

(3 set of 10 to 15 repetitions)
☐ **Arm Power II,** page 120
☐ **Tri Blaster,** page 121
☐ **Karate Kick,** page 128
☐ **Plié Press,** page 129
☐ **Hot Calves,** page 130
☐ **Strong Center,** page 131
☐ **Crunch Combo,** page 134

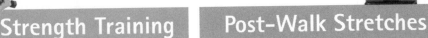

Post-Walk Stretches

☐ **Neck Stretch,** page 107
☐ **Chest & Biceps Stretch,** page 110
☐ **Triceps Stretch,** page 109
☐ **Upper Back Stretch,** page 111
☐ **Hamstring Stretch,** page 114
☐ **Quad Stretch,** page 113
☐ **Calf Stretch,** page 115

Quote of the Day
Studies indicate that the one quality all successful people have is persistence. They're willing to spend more time accomplishing a task and to persevere in the face of many difficult odds.
—Dr. Joyce Brothers

Trainer's Tip
When you stretch, there's no need to hold the position longer than 30 seconds.

245

I feel __ about my workout today:
☐ satisfied
☐ proud
☐ disappointed
☐ other _____

My goals for tomorrow:
_____
_____
_____

Part 2
Walk the Weight Away!,
Day by Day

Nutrition Guide

Suggested Menu

Breakfast

- 1 Graham Cracker Muffin (page 50)

  1 cup non-fat milk

  1 small banana

Lunch

- 1 plate Spinach Salad (page 90)

  1 handful grapes

  ½ small whole grain bagel

  1 teaspoon butter

Dinner

- 1 Oaty Beef Burger (page 63)

  1 hamburger roll

  1 small salad

  2 shakes low-fat salad dressing

Snack

1 frozen fruit juice bar

246

Walk the Weight Away!

Sweetened drinks like sodas, iced teas, and lemonades are loaded with sugar, but it's not easy to give them up cold turkey. If you want to decrease your consumption of those products, try switching to iced herbal teas. You'll find lots of varieties at your local market and you'll be surprised how good they taste with no sweetening or just a drop or two of honey.

Breakfast   time:

What I ate _____

_____

What I was doing while I ate

_____

Hunger level _____

Lunch   time:

What I ate _____

_____

What I was doing while I ate

_____

Hunger level _____

Dinner   time:

What I ate _____

_____

What I was doing while I ate

_____

Hunger level _____

Snack   time:

What I ate _____

_____

What I was doing while I ate

_____

Hunger level _____

Water

Remember to drink 8 glasses of water

I feel ___ about how I ate today:

- ☐ satisfied
- ☐ proud
- ☐ disappointed
- ☐ other _____

My goals for tomorrow:

_____

_____

_____

Workout Journal

Daily Stretches

- ☐ Head & Neck Stretch, page 107
- ☐ Shoulder Stretch, page 108
- ☐ Triceps Stretch, page 109
- ☐ Chest & Biceps Stretch, page 110
- ☐ Upper Back Stretch, page 111
- ☐ The Egg, page 112
- ☐ Quadriceps Stretch, page 113
- ☐ Hamstring Stretch, page 114
- ☐ Calf Stretch, page 115
- ☐ Butterfly Stretch, page 116

Watch the Hills

Treadmill walking is a great way to get your workout in when the weather's bad, but watch the incline. If you find you're leaning over as you walk, the incline is too steep or you're walking too fast.

Don't Let the Sunshine In

You slather yourself with sunscreen, but don't forget that your eyes need protection from the sun, too. You need sunglasses with UV protection—don't leave home without them.

Start a Walk to School Program

Build your walk into your day by organizing a neighborhood walk to school program. That way you and your kids can get exercise together.

Quote of the Day

A man's health can be judged by which he takes two at a time—pills or stairs.
—Joan Welsh

247

Part 2
Walk the Weight Away!,
Day by Day

Nutrition Guide

Suggested Menu

Breakfast

- 3 Whole Wheat Pancakes with Strawberry Syrup (page 54, page 53)

  1 cup non-fat milk

Lunch

- 1 Strawberry Orange Muffin (page 52)

  1 apple

  1 small container non-fat, no sugar added yogurt

Dinner

- 1 Pork Chop Dijon (page 74)

  ½ small sweet potato

  ½ plate steam asparagus sprinkled with lime juice

Snack

- 1 handful raw vegetables with Lemon Hummus for dipping (page 57)

248

Walk
the
Weight
Away!

Maybe you've started a healthy recipe swap with your friends. Why not start your own healthy cooking club? One way to organize it is to have several friends each prepare a healthful dinner that freezes well. Then, one night a month the group meets and divides the dinners so that each club member gets a portion of each dinner to take home and pop into the freezer.

Breakfast   time:

What I ate _____

_____

What I was doing while I ate

_____

Hunger level _____

Lunch   time:

What I ate _____

_____

What I was doing while I ate

_____

Hunger level _____

Dinner   time:

What I ate _____

_____

What I was doing while I ate

_____

Hunger level _____

Snack   time:

What I ate _____

_____

What I was doing while I ate

_____

Hunger level _____

Water

Remember to drink 8 glasses of water

I feel ___ about how I ate today:

- ☐ satisfied
- ☐ proud
- ☐ disappointed
- ☐ other _____

My goals for tomorrow:

_____

_____

_____

Workout Journal

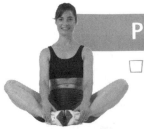

Pre-Walk Warm-Up

☐ Spend 5 to 10 minutes slowly swinging your arms to prepare for your workout.

Walking Workout

Choose one.

☐ **Distance: 3.5 miles**
(12-minute-per-mile pace)

☐ **Time: 42 min.**
(12-minute-per-mile pace)

☐ **Steps: 7000 steps**

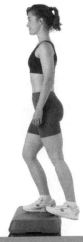

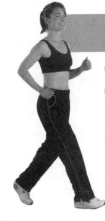

Strength Training

(3 set of 10 to 15 repetitions)

☐ **Shoulders Up,** page 118
☐ **Arm Power I,** page 119
☐ **Front Fly,** page 125
☐ **Push-Up,** page 124
☐ **Back Fly,** page 122
☐ **Thigh Shaper,** page 126
☐ **Best Butt,** page 127
☐ **Six Pack,** page 132
☐ **Basic Crunch,** page 133

Post-Walk Stretches

☐ **Neck Stretch,** page 107
☐ **Chest & Biceps Stretch,** page 110
☐ **Triceps Stretch,** page 109
☐ **Upper Back Stretch,** page 111
☐ **Hamstring Stretch,** page 114
☐ **Quad Stretch,** page 113
☐ **Calf Stretch,** page 115

I feel __ about my workout today:

☐ satisfied
☐ proud
☐ disappointed
☐ other _____

My goals for tomorrow:

_____
_____
_____

Quote of the Day
Those who think they have no time for bodily exercise will sooner or later have to find time for illness.
—Edward Stanley

Trainer's Tip
Cross-training is a great way to stay motivated, prevent boredom, and surprise your muscles. Engage in a variety of activities such as biking, swimming, and even softball.

249

Part 2
Walk the Weight Away!,
Day by Day

Nutrition Guide

Suggested Menu

Breakfast

1 small container non-fat yogurt mixed with 2 heaping tablespoons Grapenuts cereal

1 cup grapefruit juice

Lunch

• 1 ½ cups Thai Pasta Salad (page 91)

1 pear

Dinner

• ¼ plate Pork Tenderloin in Cream Sauce (page 75)

1 ear corn

¼ plate vegetable salad

2 shakes low-fat salad dressing

Snack

1 teaspoon peanut butter and 3 crackers

Just because you're pressed for time doesn't mean you can't prepare a quick, healthful dinner. Here's how: Preheat the oven to 450°F. Place one or two large sheets of heavy-duty aluminum foil on the counter. Spray the foil with a little non-fat cooking spray, and then center a 4-ounce chicken or fish fillet on the foil. Add vegetables of your choice: julienned carrots, broccoli florets, garlic. Add a tablespoon or two of lemon juice, salt and pepper to taste, and then wrap the foil to form a pouch. Bake the foil pouch for around 15 minutes, until fish or chicken is cooked through, and serve. Clean up is a snap, too.

Breakfast   time:

What I ate _____

What I was doing while I ate _____

Hunger level _____

Lunch   time:

What I ate _____

What I was doing while I ate _____

Hunger level _____

Dinner   time:

What I ate _____

What I was doing while I ate _____

Hunger level _____

Snack   time:

What I ate _____

What I was doing while I ate _____

Hunger level _____

Water

Remember to drink 8 glasses of water

I feel __ about how I ate today:
- ☐ satisfied
- ☐ proud
- ☐ disappointed
- ☐ other _____

My goals for tomorrow:
_____
_____
_____

250

Walk the **Weight** Away!

Workout Journal

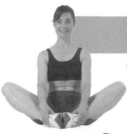

Pre-Walk Warm-Up

☐ Spend 5 to 10 minutes slowly swinging your arms to prepare for your workout.

Walking Workout

Choose one.

☐ **Distance: 4 miles**
(12-minute-per-mile pace)

☐ **Time: 48 min.**
(12-minute-per-mile pace)

☐ **Steps: 8000 steps**

Alternate Workout: 3 miles at 12-15 minute-per-mile pace)

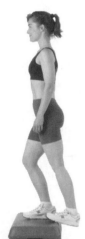
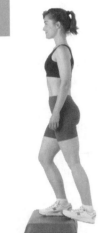

Strength Training

(3 set of 10 to 15 repetitions)
☐ **Arm Power II,** page 120
☐ **Tri Blaster,** page 121
☐ **Karate Kick,** page 128
☐ **Plié Press,** page 129
☐ **Hot Calves,** page 130
☐ **Strong Center,** page 131
☐ **Crunch Combo,** page 134

Post-Walk Stretches

☐ **Neck Stretch,** page 107
☐ **Chest & Biceps Stretch,** page 110
☐ **Triceps Stretch,** page 109
☐ **Upper Back Stretch,** page 111
☐ **Hamstring Stretch,** page 114
☐ **Quad Stretch,** page 113
☐ **Calf Stretch,** page 115

Quote of the Day
If you ever get a second chance in life for something, you've got to go all the way.
—Lance Armstrong

Trainer's Tip
Even when you're *not* on a treadmill, you may need to slow down when going up a hill or other incline; that's okay. Pick up your speed once you're back on flat ground.

I feel __ about my workout today:
☐ satisfied
☐ proud
☐ disappointed
☐ other _____

My goals for tomorrow:
_____
_____
_____

251

Part 2
Walk the Weight Away!,
Day by Day

Nutrition Guide

Suggested Menu

Breakfast

2 slices whole-grain toast

2 heaping teaspoons jam

½ pint egg substitute, scrambled

½ grapefruit

Lunch

• 1 Veggie Pita Sandwich (page 59)

1 apple

1 handful nuts

Dinner

• 1 piece Crispy Chicken (page 69)

• ¼ plate Smashed Potatoes (page 89)

• ½ plate Nutty Balsamic Green Beans (page 86)

1 individual container applesauce

Snack

6 to 8 whole grain crackers

It can be hard to appreciate how making small changes in your eating habits can add up to big results.

Eliminate this from your daily diet	*How much you'll lose in 1 year*
2 teaspoons butter on your toast	6 ¼ pounds
1 can soda	14 ½ pounds
2 teaspoons sugar in your coffee	4 pounds

Breakfast   time:

What I ate _____

_____

What I was doing while I ate

_____

Hunger level _____

Lunch   time:

What I ate _____

_____

What I was doing while I ate

_____

Hunger level _____

Dinner   time:

What I ate _____

_____

What I was doing while I ate

_____

Hunger level _____

Snack   time:

What I ate _____

_____

What I was doing while I ate

_____

Hunger level _____

Water

Remember to drink 8 glasses of water

I feel ___ about how I ate today:

☐ satisfied

☐ proud

☐ disappointed

☐ other _____

My goals for tomorrow:

_____

_____

_____

252

Walk the **Weight** Away!

Workout Journal

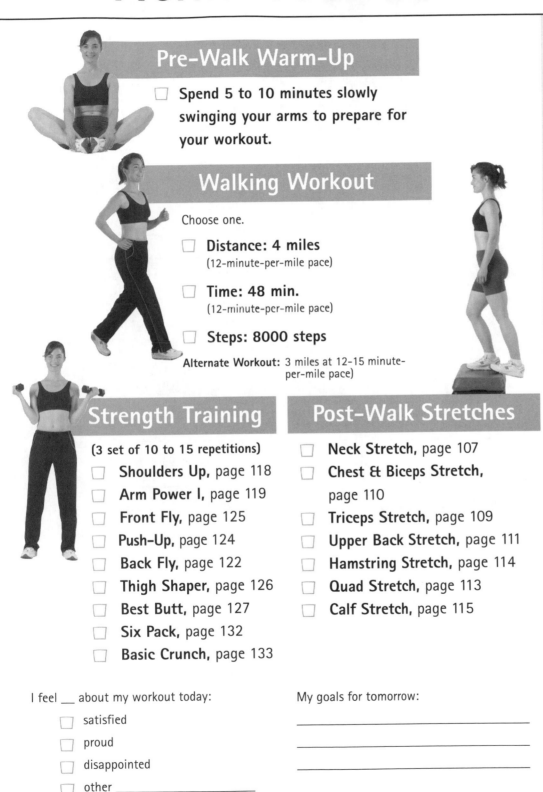

Pre-Walk Warm-Up

☐ **Spend 5 to 10 minutes slowly swinging your arms to prepare for your workout.**

Walking Workout

Choose one.

☐ **Distance: 4 miles**
(12-minute-per-mile pace)

☐ **Time: 48 min.**
(12-minute-per-mile pace)

☐ **Steps: 8000 steps**

Alternate Workout: 3 miles at 12-15 minute-per-mile pace)

Strength Training

(3 set of 10 to 15 repetitions)

☐ **Shoulders Up,** page 118
☐ **Arm Power I,** page 119
☐ **Front Fly,** page 125
☐ **Push-Up,** page 124
☐ **Back Fly,** page 122
☐ **Thigh Shaper,** page 126
☐ **Best Butt,** page 127
☐ **Six Pack,** page 132
☐ **Basic Crunch,** page 133

Post-Walk Stretches

☐ **Neck Stretch,** page 107
☐ **Chest & Biceps Stretch,** page 110
☐ **Triceps Stretch,** page 109
☐ **Upper Back Stretch,** page 111
☐ **Hamstring Stretch,** page 114
☐ **Quad Stretch,** page 113
☐ **Calf Stretch,** page 115

I feel __ about my workout today:

☐ satisfied
☐ proud
☐ disappointed
☐ other _____

My goals for tomorrow:

_____

_____

_____

Quote of the Day
Whether you think you can or you think you can't, you're right.
—Henry Ford

Trainer's Tip
Always be aware of your surroundings and the environment in which you walk.

253

Part 2
Walk the Weight Away!,
Day by Day

Nutrition Guide

Suggested Menu

Breakfast

- 1 Blueberry Muffin (page 46)

  1 small banana

  1 cup non-fat milk

Lunch

- 1 plate Spinach Salad (page 90)

  1 handful grapes

  ½ small whole grain bagel

  1 teaspoon butter

Dinner

- 1 piece Grilled Marinated Salmon (page 70)
- ¼ plate Rice Pilaf (page 87)
- ½ plate Waldorf Salad (page 92)

Snack

1 piece fresh fruit

254

Walk the Weight Away!

Sundried tomatoes add zip to many kinds of dishes, from pasta to sandwiches. But steer clear of sundried tomatoes that are sold in jars. They're usually packed in oil, which adds unnecessary fat and calories. Instead, buy the tomatoes dry and soak them in a bit of hot water to soften them up.

Breakfast   time:

What I ate _____

_____

What I was doing while I ate

_____

Hunger level _____

Lunch   time:

What I ate _____

_____

What I was doing while I ate

_____

Hunger level _____

Dinner   time:

What I ate _____

_____

What I was doing while I ate

_____

Hunger level _____

Snack   time:

What I ate _____

_____

What I was doing while I ate

_____

Hunger level _____

Water

Remember to drink 8 glasses of water

I feel ___ about how I ate today:

- ☐ satisfied
- ☐ proud
- ☐ disappointed
- ☐ other _____

My goals for tomorrow:

_____

_____

_____

Workout Journal

Daily Stretches

- ☐ Head & Neck Stretch, page 107
- ☐ Shoulder Stretch, page 108
- ☐ Triceps Stretch, page 109
- ☐ Chest & Biceps Stretch, page 110
- ☐ Upper Back Stretch, page 111
- ☐ The Egg, page 112
- ☐ Quadriceps Stretch, page 113
- ☐ Hamstring Stretch, page 114
- ☐ Calf Stretch, page 115
- ☐ Butterfly Stretch, page 116

Take Up a Hobby

 Eight weeks into the program and you probably feel like a new person! Now's the time to try some of those activities that you may have avoided because you weren't fit enough: Biking, swimming, and golf are just a few ideas.

Eliminate Stitches

In the past 8 weeks you may have experienced a side ache, or stitch, during a walk. Here are some ways to avoid and eliminate them: first, don't walk immediately after a large meal or lots of liquid. Second, when the stitch hits, breathe slowly and deeply. Finally, sometimes altering your pace—either by quickening or slowing down—eliminates a stitch.

Pad Your Shoes Carefully

It can be tempting to add over-the-counter orthotics (heel cups, arch supports, and the like) to your shoes, but be careful. You may be exchanging one problem for another, since those devices can alter your gait. If you're experiencing foot pain, head to a doctor.

Quote of the Day

A good plan is like a road map: it shows the final destination and usually the best way to get there.
—H. Stanley Judd

255

Part 2
Walk the Weight Away!,
Day by Day

Nutrition Guide

Suggested Menu

Breakfast
- 1 Graham Cracker Muffin (page 50)

   1 cup non-fat milk

   1 small banana

Lunch
- 1 cup Chunky Beef & Vegetable Soup (page 67)

   ½ bagel

   1 teaspoon butter

Dinner
- 1 piece Citrus Orange Roughy (page 68)

   ¼ plate brown rice

   ¼ plate peas

   ¼ cantaloupe

Snack
   1 cup soup

Fruit smoothies make a wonderful afternoon pick-me-up. Combine non-fat milk, a piece of fruit, and a splash of pure maple syrup in a blender and process until smooth.

For an icy smoothie, stock up on frozen strawberries and add them to the milk. Peel ripened bananas and place them in zip-lock bags in the freezer. Add a banana or two to the milk for a frosty treat.

Breakfast   time:

What I ate _____

_____

What I was doing while I ate

_____

Hunger level _____

Lunch   time:

What I ate _____

_____

What I was doing while I ate

_____

Hunger level _____

Dinner   time:

What I ate _____

_____

What I was doing while I ate

_____

Hunger level _____

Snack   time:

What I ate _____

_____

What I was doing while I ate

_____

Hunger level _____

Water

Remember to drink 8 glasses of water

I feel ___ about how I ate today:

- ☐ satisfied
- ☐ proud
- ☐ disappointed
- ☐ other _____

My goals for tomorrow:

_____

_____

_____

256

Walk the Weight Away!

Workout Journal

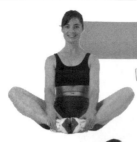

Pre-Walk Warm-Up

☐ **Spend 5 to 10 minutes slowly swinging your arms to prepare for your workout.**

Walking Workout

Choose one.

☐ **Distance: 4 miles**
(12-minute-per-mile pace)

☐ **Time: 48 min.**
(12-minute-per-mile pace)

☐ **Steps: 8000 steps**

Alternate Workout: 3 miles at 12-15 minute-per-mile pace)

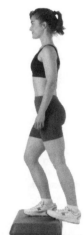
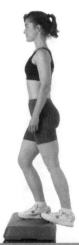

Strength Training

(3 set of 10 to 15 repetitions)
☐ **Arm Power II,** page 120
☐ **Tri Blaster,** page 121
☐ **Karate Kick,** page 128
☐ **Plié Press,** page 129
☐ **Hot Calves,** page 130
☐ **Strong Center,** page 131
☐ **Crunch Combo,** page 134

Post-Walk Stretches

☐ **Neck Stretch,** page 107
☐ **Chest & Biceps Stretch,** page 110
☐ **Triceps Stretch,** page 109
☐ **Upper Back Stretch,** page 111
☐ **Hamstring Stretch,** page 114
☐ **Quad Stretch,** page 113
☐ **Calf Stretch,** page 115

I feel __ about my workout today:
☐ satisfied
☐ proud
☐ disappointed
☐ other _____

My goals for tomorrow:

_____

_____

_____

257

Part 2
Walk the Weight Away!,
Day by Day

Nutrition Guide

Suggested Menu

Breakfast

1 small container non-fat yogurt mixed with 2 heaping tablespoons Grapenuts cereal

1 cup grapefruit juice

Lunch

- ½ plate Grilled Eggplant Wedges (page 84)

1 orange

1 handful pretzels

Dinner

- 1 bowl Pasta Primavera (page 72)

1 small vegetable salad

2 shakes low-fat dressing

1 slice Italian bread

Snack

1 low-fat bran muffin

Part of the beauty of the *Walk the Weight Away!* nutrition program is that it uses foods we're all familiar with. But that doesn't mean you can't expand your horizons; after all, variety is the spice of life. Make a point of buying a variety of fish, fruit, or vegetable that you haven't had before. Having many food options available decreases the chance of boredom.

Breakfast   time:

What I ate _____

_____

What I was doing while I ate

_____

Hunger level _____

Lunch   time:

What I ate _____

_____

What I was doing while I ate

_____

Hunger level _____

Dinner   time:

What I ate _____

_____

What I was doing while I ate

_____

Hunger level _____

Snack   time:

What I ate _____

_____

What I was doing while I ate

_____

Hunger level _____

Water

Remember to drink 8 glasses of water

I feel __ about how I ate today:

☐ satisfied
☐ proud
☐ disappointed
☐ other _____

My goals for tomorrow:

_____

_____

_____

258

Walk the Weight Away!

Workout Journal

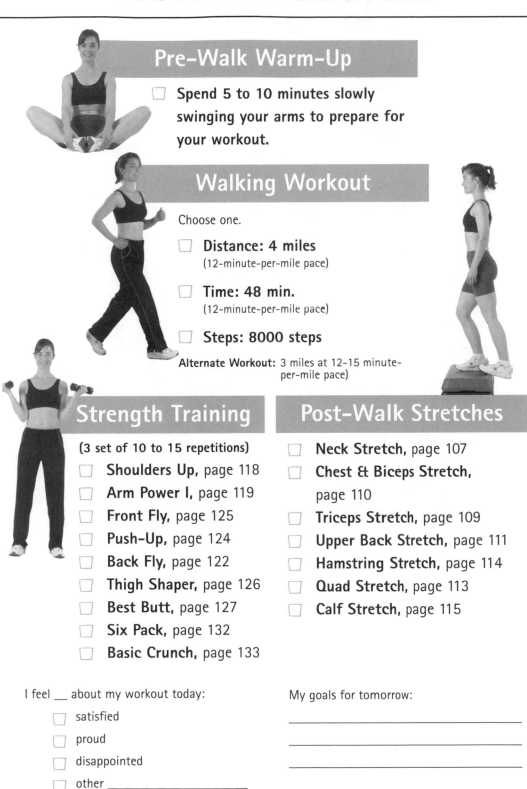

Pre-Walk Warm-Up

☐ **Spend 5 to 10 minutes slowly swinging your arms to prepare for your workout.**

Walking Workout

Choose one.

☐ **Distance: 4 miles**
(12-minute-per-mile pace)

☐ **Time: 48 min.**
(12-minute-per-mile pace)

☐ **Steps: 8000 steps**

Alternate Workout: 3 miles at 12-15 minute-per-mile pace)

Strength Training

(3 set of 10 to 15 repetitions)

☐ **Shoulders Up,** page 118
☐ **Arm Power I,** page 119
☐ **Front Fly,** page 125
☐ **Push-Up,** page 124
☐ **Back Fly,** page 122
☐ **Thigh Shaper,** page 126
☐ **Best Butt,** page 127
☐ **Six Pack,** page 132
☐ **Basic Crunch,** page 133

Post-Walk Stretches

☐ **Neck Stretch,** page 107
☐ **Chest & Biceps Stretch,** page 110
☐ **Triceps Stretch,** page 109
☐ **Upper Back Stretch,** page 111
☐ **Hamstring Stretch,** page 114
☐ **Quad Stretch,** page 113
☐ **Calf Stretch,** page 115

I feel __ about my workout today:
☐ satisfied
☐ proud
☐ disappointed
☐ other _____

My goals for tomorrow:

_____

_____

_____

Quote of the Day
Life is full of things you don't think you can do until you do them!
—Unknown

Trainer's Tip
Strive for a body weight that is healthy, not skinny.

259

Part 2
Walk the Weight Away!,
Day by Day

Nutrition Guide

Suggested Menu

Breakfast

1 small container non-fat yogurt mixed with 2 heaping tablespoons Grapenuts cereal

1 cup grapefruit juice

Lunch

- 1 ½ cups Thai Pasta Salad (page 91)

1 pear

Dinner

- 1 piece Crispy Chicken (page 69)
- ¼ plate Smashed Potatoes (page 89)
- ½ plate Nutty Balsamic Green Beans (page 86)

1 individual container applesauce

Snack

1 cup low-fat milk

260

Walk the Weight Away!

Have you ever heard that food you eat late at night is more likely to turn to fat? That's just not true. What counts is how much you eat during the day, not when you eat it. Eating late can make for an uncomfortable night, but it won't pack on pounds anymore than at any other time.

Breakfast   time:

What I ate _____

_____

What I was doing while I ate

_____

Hunger level _____

Lunch   time:

What I ate _____

_____

What I was doing while I ate

_____

Hunger level _____

Dinner   time:

What I ate _____

_____

What I was doing while I ate

_____

Hunger level _____

Snack   time:

What I ate _____

_____

What I was doing while I ate

_____

Hunger level _____

Water

Remember to drink 8 glasses of water

I feel ___ about how I ate today:

- ☐ satisfied
- ☐ proud
- ☐ disappointed
- ☐ other _____

My goals for tomorrow:

_____

_____

_____

Workout Journal

Daily Stretches

- [ ] Head & Neck Stretch, page 107
- [ ] Shoulder Stretch, page 108
- [ ] Triceps Stretch, page 109
- [ ] Chest & Biceps Stretch, page 110
- [ ] Upper Back Stretch, page 111
- [ ] The Egg, page 112
- [ ] Quadriceps Stretch, page 113
- [ ] Hamstring Stretch, page 114
- [ ] Calf Stretch, page 115
- [ ] Butterfly Stretch, page 116

Try Yoga

With all the stretching you've been doing over the last several weeks, you may be feeling flexible and loose. If you enjoy the stretching segment of your workout, you may want to look into a yoga class. Yoga helps increase overall flexibility, but it also improves posture and endurance. To find a class, check your local YMCA or YWCA. Health clubs often offer classes, too.

Have a Treat

After eight weeks of walking, you deserve a reward: Treat yourself to a foot massage!

Keep it Up!

You've reached your goal, so take some time to set new goals for the short term: Lose another pound or two, increase your speed, or enter a race. Setting goals will keep you motivated.

Quote of the Day

When we see problems as opportunities for growth, we tap a source of knowledge within ourselves which carries us through.
—Marsha Sinetar

261

Part 2
Walk the Weight Away!,
Day by Day

Nutrition Guide

How have your eating habits changed over the last eight weeks? Do you eat more fruits and vegetables? Less junk food? Are you drinking more water? In the days and weeks to come, flip through your food and workout journal and use the information it offers.

Suggested Menu

Breakfast

- 3 Whole Wheat Pancakes with Strawberry Syrup (page 54, page 53)

  1 cup non-fat milk

Lunch

- 1 Heart-Healthy Egg Salad Sandwich (page 56)

  raw cucumber slices

  1 apple

Dinner

- 1 portion Southwestern Pork Tenderloin (page 77)

  1 ear corn

  ½ plate mixed vegetable salad

  1 tablespoon low-fat salad dressing

Snack

  1 handful dried fruit

Breakfast   time:

What I ate _____

_____

What I was doing while I ate

_____

Hunger level _____

Lunch   time:

What I ate _____

_____

What I was doing while I ate

_____

Hunger level _____

Dinner   time:

What I ate _____

_____

What I was doing while I ate

_____

Hunger level _____

Snack   time:

What I ate _____

_____

What I was doing while I ate

_____

Hunger level _____

Water

Remember to drink 8 glasses of water

I feel __ about how I ate today:
- ☐ satisfied
- ☐ proud
- ☐ disappointed
- ☐ other _____

My goals for tomorrow:

_____

_____

_____

262

Walk the **Weight** Away!

Workout Journal

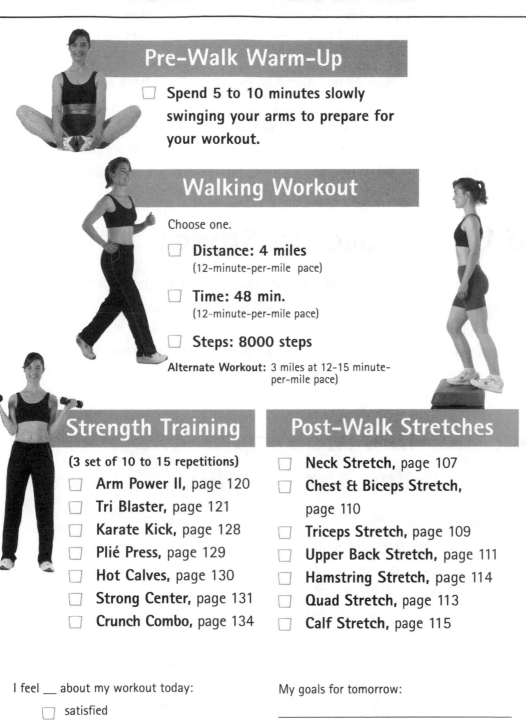

Pre-Walk Warm-Up

☐ **Spend 5 to 10 minutes slowly swinging your arms to prepare for your workout.**

Walking Workout

Choose one.

☐ **Distance: 4 miles**
(12-minute-per-mile pace)

☐ **Time: 48 min.**
(12-minute-per-mile pace)

☐ **Steps: 8000 steps**

Alternate Workout: 3 miles at 12-15 minute-per-mile pace)

Strength Training

(3 set of 10 to 15 repetitions)

☐ **Arm Power II,** page 120
☐ **Tri Blaster,** page 121
☐ **Karate Kick,** page 128
☐ **Plié Press,** page 129
☐ **Hot Calves,** page 130
☐ **Strong Center,** page 131
☐ **Crunch Combo,** page 134

Post-Walk Stretches

☐ **Neck Stretch,** page 107
☐ **Chest & Biceps Stretch,** page 110
☐ **Triceps Stretch,** page 109
☐ **Upper Back Stretch,** page 111
☐ **Hamstring Stretch,** page 114
☐ **Quad Stretch,** page 113
☐ **Calf Stretch,** page 115

I feel __ about my workout today:
☐ satisfied
☐ proud
☐ disappointed
☐ other _____

My goals for tomorrow:
_____
_____
_____

Quote of the Day

Go confidently in the direction of your dreams! Live the life you've imagined!
—Henry David Thoreau

Trainer's Tip

If you smoke, seriously consider quitting. It is the single worst thing you can do for your body. You'll find your walk more enjoyable and easier too.

263

Part 2
Walk the Weight Away!,
Day by Day

You Made It!

Congratulations on finishing the *Walk the Weight Away!* program. How do you feel? Are you pleased with the results? Take some time now to think back on how far you've come and to feel proud of all of your hard work. Also, now's the time to take an "after" picture of yourself and glue it in the back of this book alongside your "before" picture.

If you've reached your goal weight, you may want to set some new goals about how you'll maintain your success. If you still have pounds to lose, continue on the program, gradually increasing the amount of time or distance you walk.

Send Us Your Success Stories

Did you take "before" and "after" photographs of yourself while on the *Walk the Weight Away!* program? We'd love to see them and share in your success.

Attach your photographs to the space provided and label them with the date each was taken. Send the photographs to us and we'll post them on our Web site, walktheweightaway.com.

Join the *Walk the Weight Away!* on-line community:

- **Find out more** about walking for weight-loss.
- **Get answers** to your walking questions from our fitness pros.
- **Learn how to start** your own walking club.
- **Sign up** to receive a free Healthy Living e-newsletter.
- **Receive special offers** on fitness books and products.

And more!

Visit today at **www.walktheweightaway.com**

Before	After

Date: _____ | Date: _____

Name _____

Address _____

City, State, Zip Code _____

Telephone _____

Email _____

 Send your photographs to:
Walk the Weight Away!
Healthy Living Books
5–22 46th Avenue, Suite 200
Long Island City, NY 11101

Photographs become property of Healthy Living Books and cannot be returned.

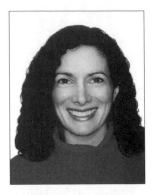

RoseMarie Alfieri is certified by the American Council on Exercise (ACE) and holds a master of arts degree in Health Education. She has written for scores of magazines and is co-author of *Combat Fat!*

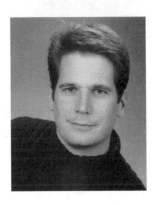

Andrew Flach is certified by the American Council on Exercise (ACE). An expert on weight management and exercise, his work has been featured on National Public Radio and in hundreds of newspapers across the country. He is the co-author of *Combat Fat!* and other popular titles on diet and exercise.

About Our Model

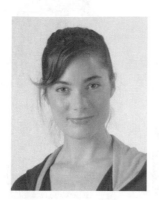

Mary Remington is a model and actress. For her, fitness is a way of life. "I am happy with my body and where I am physically," she says. "It's a goal I reach for everyday." To keep fit, Mary runs, rows, and kayaks.

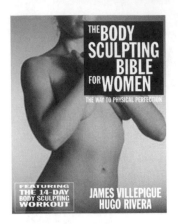
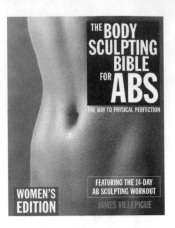
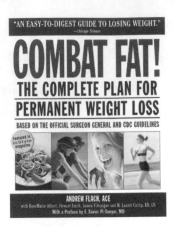

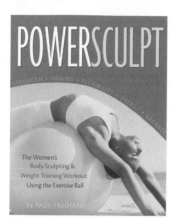
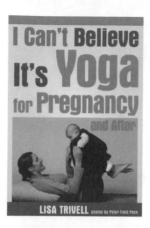
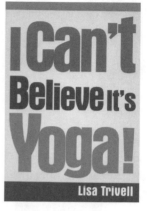
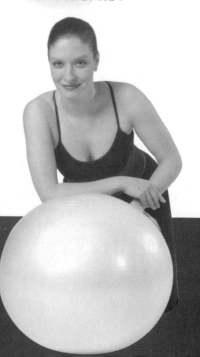

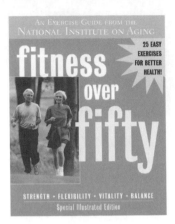
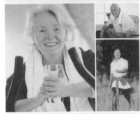
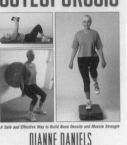
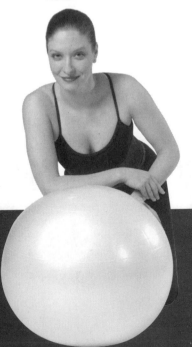

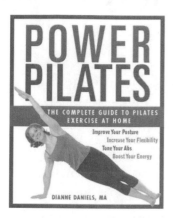
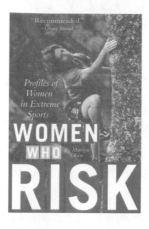
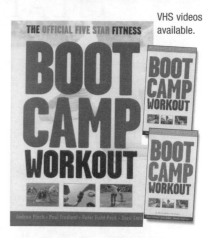

HEALTHY LIVING BOOKS

Healthy Living Books brings together recognized experts from the fields of health, medicine, fitness, and nutrition to provide millions of men and women with the reliable information they need to lead longer, healthier lives.

Our editors recognize that good health comes from healthy lifestyle choices: eating well, exercising regularly, and preventing illness through sound knowledge and intelligent action.

In this day and age, when fewer people are covered by health insurance and more face increased health risks due to sedentary lifestyles, improper nutrition, and the challenges of aging, there is a profound need for solid, tested guidance. That's where we fit in.

Our medical team consists of physicians and specialists from the country's leading medical centers and institutions. Our recipes are kitchen-tested for reliability and include nutritional analysis so that home cooks will find it easy to put delicious, healthful meals on the table. Our exercise programs are prepared by nationally certified personal trainers and rehabilitation experts. All titles are presented in clear, concise language that makes reading fun and useful.

Visit our Web site at www.healthylivingbooks.com

Healthy Living Books has something for everyone.